MANAGING

CHRONIC

PAIN

For Hugh…
Thanks for your understanding,
support and encouragement.

MANAGING CHRONIC PAIN

JEAN CRAIG

NEW HOLLAND

First published in the UK in 2003 by
New Holland Publishers (UK) Ltd
London • Auckland • Sydney • Cape Town
www.newhollandpublishers.com

Garfield House, 86–88 Edgware Road, London W2 2EA, United Kingdom
14 Aquatic Drive, Frenchs Forest, NSW 2086, Australia
218 Lake Road, Northcote, Auckland, New Zealand
80 McKenzie Street, Cape Town 8001, South Africa

10 9 8 7 6 5 4 3 2 1

ISBN 1 84330 575 5

Publishing Manager: Anouska Good
Senior Editor: Monica Ban
Designer: Karlman Roper
Illustrator: Jeff Lang
Revised Illustrations (p66, p73): Stephen Dew
UK Consultants: Dee Burrows; Ruth Day
Production: Wendy Hunt
Printer: Kyodo Printer Co (Singapore) Pte Ltd
Cover photo: photolibrary.com

*The treatments and therapies described in this book are not intended to replace the
services of trained health professionals. Your own physical condition and diagnosis
may require specific modifications or precautions. Before undertaking any treatment
or therapy, you should consult your family doctor or healthcare practitioner. Any
application of the ideas, suggestions and procedures set forth in this book are at the
reader's discretion and the author or publisher will enter into no legal liability.*

CONTENTS

ACKNOWLEDGEMENTS

My heartfelt thanks go to Lucille White, Kelly and Richard Craig who were always there with love, support, humour and encouragement. Also thanks to Dr Graham Rice, Head of the Pain Program, and his team at the Holy Spirit Rehabilitation Unit in Brisbane. And to the many people I have met over the years as hospital patients, who have shared their thoughts and feelings with me.

INTRODUCTION

As a social worker I have been employed in various hospitals around Australia. I have worked in accident and emergency departments, paediatrics (children's wards), maternity units, palliative care units, medical and surgical wards. I have often come into contact with people experiencing acute pain in hospital accident and emergency departments; individuals who have had work or motor vehicle accidents resulting in a variety of injuries. While some have been able to handle severe pain, others have asked for relief from the pain prior to the healing of their injuries. This difference in handling pain has also been observed in maternity units, where women undergoing labour experience pain in the lead up to birth. Some women would pace up and down the hospital corridors distressed by the pain they were experiencing, while other soon-to-be mothers were breathing deeply while chatting to relatives. While working with people in pain on a daily basis, I began to question, 'What is it that makes some people cope with pain while others find it difficult to manage?'

I first became aware of the answers to this question, when I began working with people who had chronic pain. My own experience of individuals with this condition was in the medical and palliative care wards of a large hospital. It was during this time, in the 1980s, that I began to do some research into the management of pain as I wanted to have something to offer patients who were experiencing it. Back then, most pain relief options were limited in comparison to what is available today. An important insight gained from reading the literature available at that time was that pain is unique to the individual who is experiencing it. My varied work experiences with children and adults, and the different injuries and illnesses experienced by these individuals indicated to me that age, sex, culture and the type of injury or illness all have to be taken into consideration when working with people in pain. For example, a pain relief method that works for an adult may not work for a child.

From my professional experiences with people in pain, I came to the conclusion that the ones who handle pain well were individuals who had knowledge about his or her illness, the skills to handle the situation and the support of healthcare professionals, family and friends.

Unfortunately, in 1995, I was diagnosed with fibromyalgia and began to experience chronic pain myself. While I had a lot of skills and experience in managing pain from a professional healthcare perspective, it is quite a different case when it happens to you. After almost a year of trying to work in a physically and mentally demanding full time position, I knew I needed some extra help to gain acceptance of a life with chronic pain. I booked myself into a pain rehabilitation programme and, while I found the physical side hard going, I gained new skills and knowledge from an individual perspective and I received encouragement and support from both the patients and staff. I left the programme knowing I had to take control and change some aspects of my life if I was going to manage my pain.

The chapters in this book are based on my professional and personal experiences of chronic pain. The book is designed to provide you with many different options to help you manage your pain – from seeking assistance from medical, surgical and allied health professionals to examining a number of alternative therapies available and looking after yourself by using the self-help section.

Body chemistry, personality and life's experiences make pain a unique and individual experience, so what is suitable for one person may not be suitable for another. Use your own good judgement when considering any of the suggestions in this book. Try things cautiously, one at a time and, if in doubt, talk things over with your family doctor. Do not expect immediate results; have patience and perseverance and work slowly towards pain management.

CHAPTER ONE

PAIN

Almost everyone in their lifetime, from childhood to old age, will be affected by pain, whether it is an injury at work, home or school, pregnancy, a premenstrual tension headache, during recovery from a surgical operation or an age-related illness such as osteoporosis or arthritis. For some of these pain-related conditions, the pain is *acute*, that is, a pain that does not last long, and, while it may be uncomfortable at the time, the pain subsides as the illness or injury improves. However, for others, particularly the aged with arthritic conditions, those with damage to the spine and those terminally ill with cancer, the pain does not diminish and becomes *chronic* over a period of time. Chronic pain is pain that persists beyond the expected healing time – it is either always present or constantly recurring. Chronic pain is thought of in medical terms as a combination of physical, mental and emotional factors that may be accompanied by an injury or illness.

Research suggests that there are several myths about chronic pain. The myth, 'it's all in your head', may have come about because, historically, doctors had no answers or treatments to offer in curing chronic pain, thus believing the pain to be a figment of the person's imagination. Unfortunately this led to the person experiencing pain to believe it was something he or she deserved for past wrongs or for abusing his or her body through the over-use of alcohol, cigarettes or drugs.

Chronic pain may be more widespread than we actually think. One only has to ask general practitioners about their caseloads involving chronic pain, or employers about the cases of absenteeism, to know how widespread the issue of pain really is. Chronic pain can also complicate the original injury or illness, with the people who are experiencing this type of pain often displaying secondary psychological symptoms, such as anxiety and depression.

Pain is an unpleasant sensory experience that is uniquely filtered through the individual's nerves, body chemistry and life activities. Pain is whatever the person experiencing it says it is. It is true that the degree of a person's pain can be controlled through activities that use the mind and this will be discussed in more detail later in the book (see Guided Imagery and Visualisation on page 92).

In a self-help guide for their patients with back pain, the Occupational Therapy Department at the Bundaberg District Health Service in Queensland, Australia suggests that pain can be felt on two levels:

- The **primary** level is where the 'sensation of pain' is sensed through the nerve endings that recognise pain in reaction to an injury. These nerve endings are called nociceptors, and are scattered throughout the body. These nociceptors transmit damage reports in the form of electrical impulses to a vast network of nerves in the peripheral nervous system. The peripheral nervous system has cranial nerves and spinal nerves that are attached to the central nervous system. The central nervous system is made up of the brain and the spinal cord and it is the nerves in the spinal cord that relay pain messages to the brain. Nerve cells in the spinal cord may also release chemicals that amplify or subdue these pain messages. Some of these chemicals produce their own painkillers (e.g. endorphins), while others (e.g. encephalin) produce 'stop pain' messages. Serotonin is a chemical that alters mood and therefore the perception of pain. There are other substances, such as a protein known as Substance P, that stimulate nerve endings and increase the pain messages.

- The **secondary** level of pain is the 'perception of pain' where the pain message radiates from deep structures in the brain to the outer cortex where it is linked with thoughts, feelings, mood, attitudes and beliefs. The brain's perception of pain moves through the

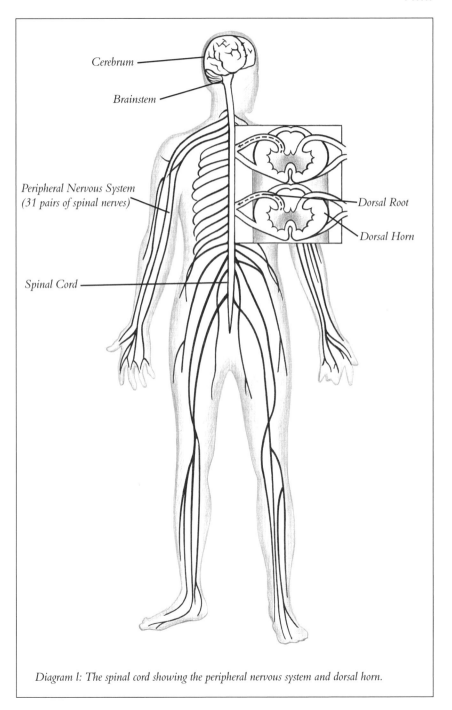

Diagram 1: The spinal cord showing the peripheral nervous system and dorsal horn.

limbic system, whose nerve fibres extend to many different areas of the brain. The limbic system also plays a part in the emotions people feel towards pain. These reactions are affected by the amygdala, displayed in Diagram 2. The emotions of sadness or unhappiness are created in the amygdala and intensify the way the cerebral cortex perceives pain messages.

The Bundaberg District Health Service also suggests that as individuals we can have an effect on the secondary level of pain perception. Pain can be increased by:
- Anticipation – the expectation of pain can produce pain
- Attention – concentrating on pain increases it
- Anxiety – anxiety tenses the muscles thus increasing our sensitivity to pain
- Anger – internalising anger results in stress and our muscle tension increases

Researchers have developed a theory about how pain occurs, which has become known as the Gate Control Theory. This theory suggests that

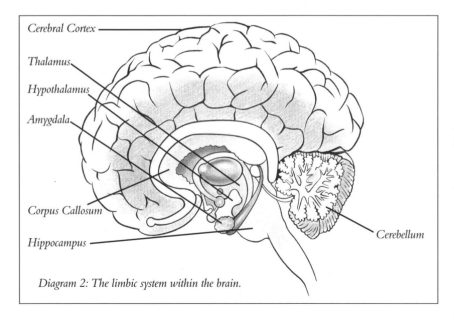

Diagram 2: The limbic system within the brain.

the dorsal columns of the spinal cord (as displayed in Diagram 1) receive sensations which they send to the brain. The dorsal horn acts as a gate to allow some painful sensations to reach the brain, depending on how their strength compares to other messages that may be attempting to reach the brain at the same time. A slight pain signal plus an added message of anxiety may be enough to open the gate, whereas the pain messages alone may not trigger the gate. The gate can be influenced by physical, mental and emotional factors. The factors that might make pain worse include:

- **Physical** – the extent of the injury or degenerative change, and residual scarring after healing and muscle tension
- **Mental** – the degree to which one focusses on pain, boredom (e.g. reduced interests and activities), beliefs and attitudes about the meaning of pain (e.g. chest pain indigestion versus heart attack), lack of control over pain (e.g. feeling helpless)
- **Emotional** – depression, anxiety, worry, tension, anger and high levels of excitement

However, researchers also suggest that this gate can be closed to reduce the amount of pain messages reaching the brain. Factors that reduce pain levels include:

- **Physical** – drugs (e.g. analgesics, sedatives, non-steroidal anti-inflammatory drugs also known as NSAIDs), counter stimulation (e.g. heat, massage and acupuncture, Transcutaneous Nerve Stimulation or TENS), and surgery
- **Mental** – distractions, such as concentrating intensely on something other than pain, having an attitude of active coping and control over pain
- **Emotional** – relaxation and stress reduction, reduced anxiety, reduced depression, increased pleasure and happiness

Chronic pain management is a process of rehabilitation and adjustment rather than a cure, and you should aim for a minimisation of the pain-related disability. The path to pain control is a direction, an attitude, a way of looking at your life and your pain that will lead you to feel less pain and be better able to cope with any you do feel. Diagram 3 shows how chronic pain can become both negative and self-destructive.

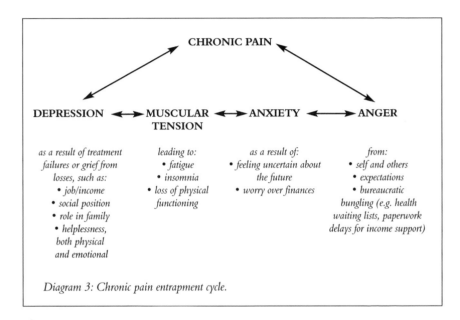

Diagram 3: Chronic pain entrapment cycle.

Your own struggle with chronic pain will have given you a wealth of knowledge and individual expertise that a good number of the healthcare professionals are not aware of. This is not meant to dismiss professional help, as healthcare professionals can teach you new skills and provide you with useful information to manage your pain. You, in turn, can provide them with your personal experiences and observations of *living* with chronic pain. Recognition of what your personal needs are to assist you in managing your pain can provide you with the key to gaining control over your pain when seeking assistance from healthcare professionals. There is more information on the role of different healthcare professionals in relation to pain management in Chapter Four (see pages 32–43).

CHAPTER TWO

COMMON MEDICAL CONDITIONS INVOLVING CHRONIC PAIN

There are certain medical ailments in which chronic pain is part of the condition and the following information on some of the more common pain-related illnesses has been included for those people who feel they may not have knowledge on their particular condition. The list is by no means exhaustive and if your medical condition is not listed here then refer to your family doctor to obtain more information.

ANGINA

Angina is a common type of heart disease that occurs when some part of the heart does not receive an adequate supply of oxygen-rich blood because the blood vessels that feed it are blocked. There are lifestyle factors that can cause our arteries to become blocked, such as high cholesterol levels from eating too many fats and sugars in our daily diet, a sedentary lifestyle without regular exercise, and high blood pressure from stress that silts up the artery walls. When the arteries that lead to the heart are diseased they become narrowed and cannot give the required amount of oxygen, thus causing pain.

Angina feels like a squeezing or gripping sensation in the centre of the chest, sometimes spreading to the shoulder, up the neck and down the arm. This pain is intermittent in nature and not present all of the time. Symptoms of angina are breathlessness which tends to subside on resting, fatigue or a feeling of tiredness and limbs that feel heavy. Rest is prescribed during an angina attack and you have probably been advised to take your angina medication the instant you have an attack. The nitrate group of drugs that are usually prescribed for angina work very quickly once you place the tablet(s) or use the spray under your tongue during an attack. Beta-blockers are another form of medication, which are very effective in reducing the frequency of angina attacks. From research into heart disease, family doctors now suggest that a daily dose of aspirin can work as a preventative measure for angina, but should not be used without medical advice. Panic or fear seems to exacerbate the pain levels in an angina attack, so it is important to deal with these emotions. Emotional self-help is discussed elsewhere (see page 83).

ARTHRITIS

Arthritis is a disease characterised by swollen and inflamed joints. There are over one hundred different forms but there are two common types – rheumatoid arthritis and osteoarthritis.

Rheumatoid arthritis is a chronic disease very common amongst our aging population, although there are numbers of young adolescents who also suffer from it. Rheumatoid arthritis affects the body's immune system. The immune system attacks the joints, causing inflammation to the joints, which then become painful and swollen. Over time there is damage to the cartilage that may result in joint deformities. Joints attacked in rheumatoid arthritis tend to be the hands, feet and knees. Joint stiffness in the morning or after inactivity, muscle weakness and fatigue because of the inability to sleep through the pain from the joints, are symptoms of this disease.

Osteoarthritis is caused by the breakdown of cartilage inside certain joints, such as those found in the neck, fingers, lower back, hips and knees, of which the latter two seem to be the most susceptible to degeneration. In the early stages of osteoarthritis the articular cartilage becomes pitted.

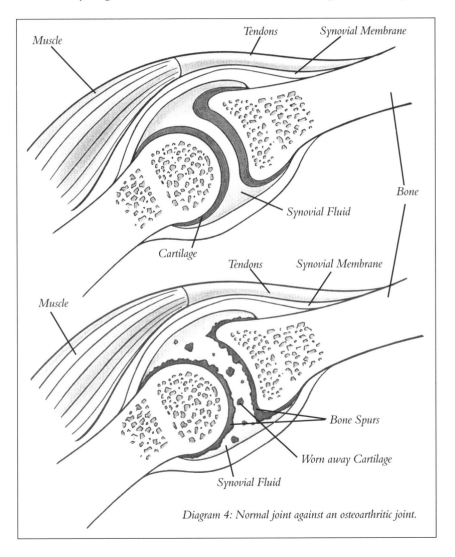

Diagram 4: Normal joint against an osteoarthritic joint.

There may be some pain and stiffness at this stage and some inflammation of the synovial membrane may occur. In the later stages of osteoarthritis, erosion of the cartilage has advanced to expose raw bone. Cartilage acts as a cushion between the bones and as it erodes away, inflammation and swelling occur and there is pain and stiffness on movement. Degeneration of the joint cartilage appears to be part of the aging process, as almost 90 per cent of people over the age of 60 show some form of osteoarthritis.

Speak to anyone with arthritis and they will tell you that chronic pain is part of this medical condition. However, it is not always severe pain but a pain that is always present on differing levels. Those who have had arthritis over a long period of time may have adjusted their lifestyle to include adequate exercise and leisure activities, a good diet, and balanced work, rest and relaxation.

BACK PAIN

Back pain affects many Western people. The major causes appear to be from an injury or an accumulation of stress on the back over a number of years (i.e. poor posture, poor fitness, poor lifting, stress and lifestyle).

Needless to say that alleviating back pain usually rests on medication and reversing accumulated habits. This involves being aware of how we stand, sit and lift and to change our posture to relieve the pressure we are putting on our lower back. It is widely believed that exercise designed to the individual's particular back problem can assist in relieving the problems of poor posture, fitness or lifestyle habits.

The herniation of discs, osteoarthritis of the vertical joints and spondylosis cause lower back pain in less than one-third of cases. Herniation of a disc is where the disc pushes itself out of its space and presses on a nerve root. About 60 per cent of people are helped by surgery to remove a disc when it is clearly causing nerve root compression.

Spondylosis often occurs in conjunction with osteoarthritis and bad posture exacerbates this disease. Bending forwards to lift or sitting too long and some types of exercise all seem to exacerbate the pain. Those

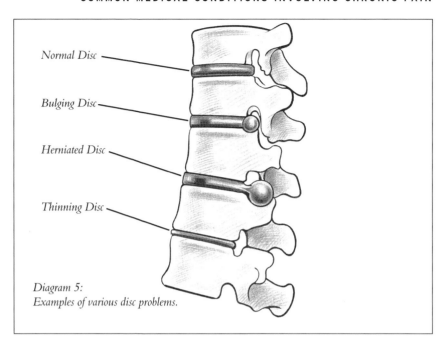

Normal Disc

Bulging Disc

Herniated Disc

Thinning Disc

Diagram 5:
Examples of various disc problems.

who experience pain in this regard often find comfort in having the body upright, either standing or lying down straight on their back.

Lower back pain is usually unpleasant as it is deep, aching, burning or shooting and sometimes immobilises the person who is terrified of triggering a severe bout of pain. Shooting pain down the leg is called sciatic pain because it follows the pattern of the sciatic nerves. This bundle of nerves runs from the lower back through the legs to the feet. Sciatic pain is often the result of disc problems.

It is possible that the major culprit in many cases of lower back pain is abnormal activity in the nerve root fibres due to minor changes in the surrounding vertebrae and tissues. The roots may be affected by compression caused by degenerative disc material, which commonly appears with aging, interference with the blood supply or stress on the ligaments and joints that surround the nerve.

Back pain affects many people and, judging by what they have to say about their back pain, it is fair to assume they experience chronic pain on differing levels. These people experience days of reduced activity due to back pain and days where they can complete their normal daily tasks.

CANCER

In terminal/end-stage cancer, the pain often stems from a tumour pressing against the bones and other tissues or interfering with the blood flow needed for the functioning of the organs. Pain can also come from cancer growths on the nerves. Unfortunately the overwhelming emotions that accompany this particular disease, such as fear, anxiety or depression, tend to aggravate the severity of the pain.

Radiation is a method used to treat certain types of cancer. Its purpose is to destroy cancerous cells and damage the blood cells that nourish the tumour. Radiation may produce scarring that can trap the nerves and pain may result from this. There are also people who experience post-operative pain as a result of the removal of tumours. Chemotherapy is another treatment where the person receives anticancer drugs to eradicate existing cancer cells or to impede the growth of new cancer cells.

Medication plays a predominant role in the management of pain from cancer. It has been suggested that the use of simple analgesics (e.g. paracetamol) is effective, safe and inexpensive. If the pain is moderate and paracetamol no longer controls the pain then codeine, which is a little stronger, may well have more effect in controlling the pain. Drugs such as morphine, a strong opioid, are used in end stage cancer. While medication plays an important part in the pain management of this disease, many of the options listed in this book for pain relief are used throughout the period of the illness, both as a means of relieving intermittent pain and in addressing the issues of anxiety the person may be experiencing.

FIBROMYALGIA

Fibromyalgia is a form of muscular rheumatism. Unlike arthritis, which targets the joints, fibromyalgia targets muscles, tendons and ligaments – there is no inflammation, just pain. When diagnosing fibromyalgia, medical specialists in rheumatology look for a certain number of tender points within the body, which are painful under slight pressure.

The main symptom of fibromyalgia is 'aching all over', similar to that experienced during episodes of the flu, but much more severe. Other symptoms include difficulty sleeping, stiffness, sensitivity to weather changes and headaches. Fibromyalgia is thought to be a syndrome because there are other illnesses involved, such as circulatory problems, irritable bowel syndrome, cognitive problems and chronic fatigue.

Fibromyalgia does not have a cure. Factors like stress, poor sleep and physical or emotional trauma can trigger moderate to severe episodes of the illness. Research suggests immune system abnormalities, such as a lack of cortisol (a hormone that controls the level of immune system activity), occur in people with fibromyalgia. This lack of cortisol leads to an overactive immune system that attacks the body. Other research has pointed to chemical imbalances, such as a lack of serotonin in the brain. Giving people with fibromyalgia anti-depressants (which increase the amount of serotonin) has led to a reduction in symptoms. Yet other research shows that people with fibromyalgia have a high level of Substance P, a protein that stimulates nerve endings and causes pain.

Fibromyalgia pain has been described as burning, throbbing, stabbing, shooting or just a deep gnawing ache. The pain may be worse in one particular area of the body. Research suggests that back pain and headaches are the most common forms of fibromyalgic pain experienced. The tender point test used by rheumatologists when diagnosing the illness indicates that pain can be experienced at different sites throughout the body.

MIGRAINE

Migraine headaches are much more intense than tension type headaches; they not only grab your attention but can also put your life on hold because they can last from a few hours to a few days. With migraines, there is a throbbing pain caused by spasms of the blood vessels around the brain, usually on one side of the head, accompanied by nausea or vomiting. Loud noise or bright lights may intensify the pain. Some people experience a loss of vision or vision that is clouded by black spots. Others may experience an aura.

One of the causes suggested is an imbalance of the brain chemistry. Migraines may also be hereditary. They affect far more women than men. Diet, as in reactions to certain foods, is another theory for what causes migraines. This is discussed later in the book (see page 33). Stress, particularly when one is tense and/or frustrated, is also thought to be another cause of migraines. Other research suggests that environmental factors such as sunlight or changes in the weather may also trigger migraine attacks. Yet other factors suggest that migraines in some women can be caused by taking the contraceptive pill or from hormonal replacement therapy in menopausal women.

MULTIPLE SCLEROSIS

Many people with Multiple Sclerosis (MS) experience pain even though it is often thought of as a pain-free disease. Spasms, altered muscle balance and nerve damage cause the pain, which often increases with age. Muscle pain can be aching and mild or moderate. Nerve pain is often described as pins and needles, or burning. It can be made worse by heat and tiredness and it can also get worse when you first lie down to rest. Usually the intensity wears off after a little while. Medications, such as Amitriptyline, can help the pain as well as some of the other techniques in the book.

PHANTOM LIMB PAIN

Some people who have had a limb amputated speak of feeling sensations (i.e. itching or burning) coming from the missing limb. This indicates that the brain is still receiving messages from the severed nerve fibres and is interpreting the messages as if the limb were still present. Many say that the sensations lessen over time, while others say they experience sensation and pain (i.e. stabbing, shooting and/or throbbing). Research into phantom limb pain suggests that people who had pain in the limb prior to the amputation may experience more pain than those who had no pain before the amputation. Other research suggests that people who lose their limb in an accident may experience more pain than those who have planned surgery. Amputations can occur as a result of many things including injury, cancer or diabetes.

SHINGLES

Shingles is caused by the same virus that causes chicken pox. Instead of the spots one gets with chicken pox, shingles is a painful rash that eventually erupts into clusters of pus-filled blisters. The earlier you get to see your family doctor, the shorter the course of the illness. Antiviral drugs are prescribed during the acute phase and when the blisters have healed, Axacin, an ointment that contains capsaicin (the substance that makes pepper hot), can be used. This ointment will reduce the chemical Substance P, and acts on nerve endings to dull the sensation of pain. Some people may find the ointment itself causes a burning sensation on the skin. It can be used up to four times a day and, because it can have a delayed action, you may need a couple of weeks to fully assess its benefits.

In some cases the pain can be shooting or burning and the skin becomes highly sensitive to the slightest touch. Clothing or a change in temperature can trigger the pain. Light, loose fitting clothes are much more comfortable to wear during an attack of shingles. It is thought that the shingles rash is associated with the inflammation of nerves beneath the skin. Shingles usually follows the path of the inflamed nerve from the middle of the chest to the middle of the back, down one side of the body. Sometimes the rash may reach the face, where care should be taken to stop it reaching the eyes, as it may affect the sight. Suspected triggers to the rash can be stress, injury or a temporary weakness in the immune system. Shingles is less infectious than chicken pox because the virus is not airborne, but care should be taken as the virus can be transmitted with close contact, and cause chicken pox (but not shingles) in someone who has not had chicken pox before. Shingles pain may progress to post-herpetic neuralgia, which is a complex chronic pain, and your family doctor may suggest specialist management.

WHIPLASH

This sometimes occurs following a car accident. You may get pain in your neck and shoulders that can last a long time. Sometimes it is the muscles being bruised and tense. Occasionally a nerve may be trapped or inflamed. You may have to have a neck collar at the time of injury to wear for a week or so. Research shows that long term use of these is not helpful. Whiplash is usually treated with simple painkillers and physiotherapy. However, it can become a chronic pain and many of the suggestions in the book may be helpful.

When you experience life with pain, firstly see your family doctor to see if a medical diagnosis can be made as to the cause of the pain. It may be one of the conditions described in this chapter, something else, or the doctors may not be able to put a name to it. Discuss the treatment options with your doctor.

CHAPTER THREE

MEDICAL AND SURGICAL OPTIONS FOR PAIN MANAGEMENT

The key to living with chronic pain is understanding what can be done to keep the pain at an acceptable/manageable level so you can get on with your life. This involves seeking a medical opinion and can include undergoing various medical tests to provide you with a diagnosis if this is possible.

MEDICAL OPTIONS

What is involved in finding out a medical diagnosis? For you, it is a trip to your family doctor, where you will need to explain your medical history and the symptoms you are currently experiencing. The doctor will conduct a medical examination based on the symptoms you have described. It may well be that further tests will be required (see page 26) or it may be that your family doctor will treat your pain. Occasionally, your doctor may write out a referral for you to see a specialist in relation to your symptoms. For example:

- Anaesthetist – who specialises in treating chronic pain
- Back Pain Specialist – this could be an orthopaedic surgeon or a physiotherapist
- Cardiologist – for angina and chest pain
- Neurologist or Neurosurgeon – for nerve-related problems such as multiple sclerosis, headaches and some back pains
- Oncologist – for cancer pain and treatments
- Orthopaedic surgeon – for joint replacement
- Psychologist – for support in managing all types of pain
- Rheumatologist – for arthritis, fibromyalgia and back pain

Blood tests

Your family doctor or specialist may suggest you have some blood tests. These may say something about your general health or about a possible cause for your pain. Ask your doctor or specialist what your test is for.

X-rays and scans

There are various x-rays and scans that may help to diagnose your condition. Following is a brief description of them:

- X-rays are radioactive pictures, which can, for example, show arthritic and degenerative changes in the joints and vertebrae.
- Magnetic Resonance Imaging (MRI) scan is a way of getting a picture of the inside of your body. The test is most useful for finding abnormalities in the brain, spinal cord, bones, joints, heart and other organs.
- Bone scans involve having a radioactive chemical injected into the bloodstream. This chemical attaches itself to areas of bone that are undergoing rapid change and show up as dark patches on the radiographic pictures.
- Computerised Axial Tomography (CAT) scan is similar to, but more thorough than, an x-ray as it gives a three-dimensional

view of inside the body. It is less commonly used now that MRI is available.

- Other more specialised tests may be requested by the specialist.

A diagnosed illness can provide you with a number of answers as to why you have pain and the treatment options available for your medical condition. However, it is useful for you to know that any diagnosis may differ between medical personnel. The reasons for these differences in medical opinion are often because of similarities in symptoms in some conditions. For example, symptoms of marked pain and morning joint stiffness on initial presentation to a rheumatologist could either be fibromyalgia or polymyalgia rheumatica. After a trial of Prednisolone (a steroid medication) the diagnosis becomes more obvious as Prednisolone makes no difference to the pain of fibromyalgia. If you are faced with two different diagnoses, try to get your hands on as much information as you can (i.e. reading material and internet sources) – preferably compiled by qualified professionals – about the different diagnoses you have been given. By comparing your own symptoms and observations of daily living (i.e. what works and what does not), your own experiences will assist you with managing your pain.

Medication

When given a diagnosis by your doctor or medical specialist, you will also need to be fully informed on the factors relating to the medical condition, such as its causes, treatments and prognosis (the medical term for how long the condition will last). Seeing your family doctor for pain usually means that you will leave the surgery with a prescription for medication. You may have tried over-the-counter painkillers to relieve pain yourself before your visit to the doctor. Medication as a way of relieving pain is only one of the options available.

There are some complex issues in the use of medication, such as the various potential side-effects from different types of medicines. While the medication may be beneficial in alleviating or reducing your level of pain, it is not going to help you in the future if you damage your kidneys from over-use of an aspirin-based medication or you develop ulcers from anti-inflammatory drugs. So remember to ask your doctor what the side-effects are from the medicines that he or she is prescribing you.

Often after taking a medicine for a long period of time, it may no longer have as positive or beneficial an effect as when you first started taking it. This may mean your body has developed a tolerance to it in the prescribed amount. If this is occurring, you will need to ask your doctor whether you should take a higher dose or whether you need a different type of medication to combat your symptoms. Do not take extra medication in the belief that taking more than has been prescribed will work more effectively, as some medications are dangerous when taken in large amounts. Medications for pain come in a number of different forms:

- Capsules – e.g. Gabapentin and Celebrex
- Creams – e.g. Axacin, Movelat
- Injections – e.g. gold, opioids, Cortisone
- Liquids – e.g. Oromorph
- Patches – e.g. Transtec, Fentanyl or GTN
- Sprays – e.g. GTN
- Suppositories – e.g. Diclofenac
- Tablets – e.g. Paracetamol, Ibuprofen and Amitriptyline

Pain clinics and pain management programmes

Your family doctor may refer you to a pain clinic. The majority of NHS hospitals and some private hospitals have these as out-patient clinics. A consultant runs the pain clinic and may also have other people working with them (see page 26). At the pain clinic you may have medicines or injections prescribed for you to try and control your pain (see page 27 and above). A number of pain clinics offer complementary therapies such as acupuncture.

The pain clinic may also run a pain management programme. In some hospitals this is offered as an in-patient programme where people stay for a period of four weeks. More than often they are offered as a day a week for several weeks. A variety of healthcare professionals will help you and the other people on the pain management programme to:

- Understand your chronic pain
- Learn and practise gentle exercises
- Manage your own medication correctly
- Learn techniques to help change the spotlight from your pain to something else
- Relax in different ways
- Pace your activities
- Manage the changes in mood that chronic pain can cause
- Get the best out of your relationships with family and friends
- Take control of your pain

Some pain management programmes also have a vocational element – looking hard at getting people back into the workplace and helping them to keep their jobs.

There are some pain management programmes run by individuals – for instance the Self-Management Programme run by Pete Moore and David Matthews (see page 59 and Addresses section, page 102).

SURGICAL OPTIONS

If, having looked at your x-rays and scans, your doctor or specialist thinks you may benefit from seeing a surgeon, a referral is given to you to see an orthopaedic surgeon or a neurosurgeon for further assessment. These practitioners may perform surgery to alleviate or relieve pain.

Some of the surgical procedures to relieve pain include:

- Arthrodesis – the fusion of a joint to relieve pain and counteract instability.
- Arthroscopy – minor surgery where a small telescope is inserted into the joint to remove any loose fragments that may be grinding against the bone and causing pain.
- Discectomy – a surgical procedure for the removal of a herniated disc to relieve pressure on a nerve root.

- Laminectomy – a surgical procedure, generally performed to reduce pressure on the spinal cord and nerve roots. This allows more room for nerves of the spine and reduces the irritation and inflammation on the spinal nerves. In addition, bone spurs that may have grown around the nerves can be removed.
- Replacement surgery and total hip and knee replacement surgery – usually reserved for people with osteoarthritis when all other conventional treatments have failed. With the development of new synthetic materials, total joint replacement surgery has become a practical solution for advanced osteoarthritis as well as other conditions, such as sports injuries. The ball and socket joint in the hip, which carries most of the body weight and is essential for walking, is replaced with a duplicate made of plastic and stainless steel. The entire knee can also be replaced with a mechanical implant. Replacement surgery can reduce a person's level of disability.
- Spinal fusion – placing a bone graft between two or more vertebrae so they grow together or fuse. Bone is usually taken from the pelvic area at the time of surgery and inserted between the vertebrae.
- Sympathectomy – the surgery to remove autonomic nerves to relieve causalgia (pain that produces a burning sensation caused from damage to a peripheral nerve).

Surgery for relieving pain (particularly back pain) is often a last resort, as the success rate is unpredictable.

Anaesthetists

Anaesthetists are doctors who work with surgeons in their surgical procedures and also play a role in helping relieve people's pain. There are various specialised injections that they can perform, including:

- Epidural – a spinal injection that blocks the gateway of pain to the brain. Because it is both a complicated and specialised procedure, epidurals are performed by anaesthetists who know which part of the spine to inject and what drugs to use. Epidurals are given to pregnant women when in labour to relieve the pain of giving birth.

- Nerve blocks – where an anaesthetist injects a local anaesthetic around a nerve fibre to block its function. If its energy is blocked, the nerve message is interrupted and does not reach the brain. This procedure reduces pain in the muscle, reduces inflammation and swelling and relaxes the muscle that is producing spasms. Acute flare-ups of pain or cancer are the most common reasons for these injections.

- Trigger point injections – trigger points are tender areas often in muscles, ligaments or tendons. Pain may radiate from the points to other areas. For example, people who have a poor posture may have back pain that is also causing a secondary pain to other areas of the body. Injections, usually containing lidocaine, another local anaesthetic or steroids (an anti-inflammatory), can be given to help relieve pain.

Injections as a method of pain relief can be effective as they go straight to the root of the pain, however, you may need to be prepared to have more than one, as sometimes a course of injections tends to keep the pain at bay longer.

CHAPTER FOUR

THE ROLES OF HEALTHCARE PROFESSIONALS IN THE TREATMENT OF CHRONIC PAIN

Expanding your field of healthcare professionals to support you in the management of your chronic pain is something that can widen your knowledge and expertise, while providing you with a holistic model of healthcare.

When consulting a healthcare professional, it is important to ensure you use only those who are fully qualified in their field.

This chapter clarifies what types of assistance different healthcare professionals will be able to offer you in the management of your chronic pain. No particular healthcare professional is more important than another. The professionals cited in this chapter are listed in alphabetical order.

DIETICIANS

Weight is an important factor when faced with chronic pain, that is, maintaining a healthy weight for your height. Being overweight increases chronic pain as it overtaxes the joints. It is far too easy when chronic pain prevails to become sedentary and exclude any form of exercise, for example using the car for short distances or comfort eating out of boredom and depression. When this occurs, weight gain is inevitable. Certain medications for pain can cause weight gain as a side-effect. If this is the case, discuss with your family doctor the alternatives to this particular medication. Being overweight puts more strain on the joints thereby increasing pain levels, so an appointment to see a dietician makes good sense. The NHS has dieticians in most hospitals that carry an out-patient caseload. You will need a referral from your doctor to see one. There are a few dieticians practising privately who can be contacted via the British Dietetic Association.

Dieticians are educated in the components of different foods and can guide you in a weight maintenance programme through a healthy, nutritious diet. Studies have found that some foods and substances may increase your pain, such as alcohol, avocado, bacon, aged cheeses, chocolate, coffee, cola drinks, cold meats, herring, hot dogs, mono-sodium glutamate (MSG – an additive found in many Asian/Chinese foods), nuts, pork, red wine, sausages, smoked meats, tea, tobacco and yeast products (freshly baked).

It has long been accepted in medical/health fields that oranges, cheeses, chocolates and red wine can trigger a migraine attack. On the positive side, people suffering from arthritis have improved after eating fresh vegetables (e.g. leafy greens, celery), a good helping of fish (which contains Omega 3 oils) and freshly ground black pepper. Turkey and bananas have been found to increase levels of tryptophan (an amino acid) in people with fibromyalgia, assisting them in better sleep cycles. Research also suggests that people who have high cholesterol and blocked arteries should stick to a low-fat vegetarian diet and take mild exercise in order to allow their arteries to clean out accumulated plaque, thereby reversing blockage.

Information on tonics and pick-me-ups for those who are feeling constantly fatigued or lethargic can also be obtained from dieticians. Dieticians are able to assist you in monitoring your weight levels in proportion to your height and build. This is not only important for those people who are overweight, but also for those who are underweight and malnourished.

NURSES

Nurses are involved in a variety of chronic pain settings, such as:

- Acupuncture Clinics – some nurses are trained acupuncturists.
- At Work – Occupational Health Nurses can advise on matters affecting your pain and employment.
- In the Community – District Nurses and Macmillan Nurses may support you in your medication management, provide you with advice on alternative coping strategies and also refer you to other agencies.
- Pain Clinics – where they may advise on TENS, for example, or teach relaxation.
- Pain Management Programmes – where Nurse Specialists may offer support and advice about medication management, pacing and sexual activity.

OCCUPATIONAL THERAPISTS

Occupational therapists are healthcare professionals who can assist you in adjusting your lifestyle in order to reduce the impact of your disability. The lifestyle issues they consider include whether you work or stay at home, your social/leisure activities and your personal pursuits. Occupational therapists are also trained to make hand/finger splints for people who have hand/finger injuries or illnesses, such as repetitive strain injury (RSI) or rheumatoid arthritis. The splints in the latter case may assist in preventing further deformity of the patient's hand and fingers. For people with repetitive strain injury, the splints may help them by supporting the hands to enable them to continue working. Hand splints are appliances which are individually designed to relieve pain and inflammation by giving support to the affected joints. Occupational therapists also make braces for sufferers of carpel tunnel syndrome, which is a painful nerve compression in the wrist that can numb the fingers. Wearing a brace supports the wrist, relieves the pressure and allows the nerve to heal.

Occupational therapists have an extensive knowledge of the type of independent living aids that are available to help you be comfortable in the tasks of daily living, for example, back pain and its effects on lifting and carrying, how to get out of bed in the morning when you are stiff and sore, the type of chair that best meets your needs and how to sit down and get up from a chair. By enabling you to conserve energy in this way, occupational therapists can help you to get on with the things you want to do. They will help you pace your activities so you can lead a more normal life.

As well as working in NHS hospitals, occupational therapists carry out work with social services in the community. In their involvement with social services, occupational therapists provide advice on housing for people with disabilities, such as the width of doorways in a dwelling for a person in a wheelchair, the installation of handrails in the shower and toilet for the physically frail, or the installation of flip taps in the bathroom, laundry and kitchen for those with arthritis. Occupational therapists may visit you in your home or workplace to assess how to help you with your daily living needs. The College of Occupational Therapy keeps a list of private practitioners.

PHARMACISTS

As previously mentioned, medicines, whether they have been prescribed or bought over-the-counter, can pose their own problems. It is therefore worthwhile developing a good relationship with your pharmacist. The principles of good practice, as set out by The Royal Pharmaceutical

Society of Great Britain, require that your pharmacist explain the medication your doctor has prescribed for you and any side-effects of which you need to be aware.

Pharmacists have manuals of all the medicines that are dispensed in the UK, which explain the drug, the dosage the drug comes in and whether the drug is produced in a tablet, capsule, liquid, suppository, skin preparation or injection form. Pharmacists are also able to interpret how and when the drug should be taken and how the drug will interact with any other medication you may be taking. The pharmacist may also be able to save you money by advising whether there is a similar medication to the one prescribed by your doctor, at a lower cost. (This cheaper medication is known as a generic brand.)

These days, pharmacists not only deal in medications but are also able to help you hire or purchase living aids. These include a number of kitchen gadgets you can buy to make life easier, such as jar openers, tin openers, and cutlery with reinforced grips to make them easier to handle, for example. You can even purchase the flexible gripping by the metre to fit to your own cutlery.

Have you ever stood in a queue at the bank wishing you could sit down without losing your place? Did you know that some of the walking frames available not only have wheels for easy manoeuvrability but also have seats to sit on and that you can get walking sticks that are three-pronged and open out to carry a small seat? Provided you are not overweight, the latter may be the answer to waiting in long queues, as they are portable and fold up.

Pharmacists also sell orthopaedic shoes and orthopaedic shoe inserts for people who have aching or painful knees, backs or heels.

PHYSIOTHERAPISTS

Physiotherapists offer a range of services designed to help you keep mobile while looking after your bones, limbs and joints. Physiotherapists can advise you on an exercise programme for your particular injury or illness. Why is it important to exercise? You must have heard the slogan 'Use it or Lose it'. Physiotherapists will tell you that exercise helps keep your joints flexible and will help you to maintain strength in the muscles. Exercise may also help you regain lost flexibility – it certainly reduces the risk of deformity.

You should exercise every day. However, if you are someone who has not exercised regularly in the past, you should ensure that you start any exercise programme slowly, building up the time and repetitions as you progress.

Whenever you are about to embark on a new exercise programme it is very important to remember the rules of stretching exercises. These rules are:

- Warm up prior to stretching
- Stretch before and after exercise
- Stretch gently and slowly, then hold each stretch for between ten and fifteen seconds
- Never bounce or stretch rapidly
- Stretch to the point of tension/discomfort, NEVER pain
- Do not hold your breath while stretching

There are other exercise programmes that your physiotherapists may suggest, including:

- Gym programmes that teach you how to use the different types of gym equipment in order to provide you with suitable exercise and boost your fitness. Physiotherapists specialising in sports medicine are in favour of this type of exercise. You can get an exercise referral to your local sports centre from your family doctor or your NHS physiotherapist.
- Hydrotherapy programmes that involve performing gentle exercises in a heated swimming pool. This type of exercise is a great help to people who are troubled by stiffness and soreness from arthritis, or who suffer from back pain. The warm water assists flexibility and movement, and encourages and strengthens weak muscles. You do not have to be able to swim in order to participate in hydrotherapy, as all the exercises are performed in shallow water.

Physiotherapists can also advise you when to use hot and cold treatments to ease pain. Application of heat to sore joints gives relief when joints are stiff. Heat treatment in the home can include hot water bottles, heat packs warmed in the microwave, infrared lamps, electric blankets and warm baths or showers. Hot water bottles should not be put directly onto the skin but wrapped in a warm damp towel for a combination of moisture and heat to soothe the painful area. Cold packs can be used on hot, tender inflamed joints. Whether you use ice cubes, a commercially bought ice pack or a packet of frozen peas, never put them straight onto the inflamed area; always make sure they are wrapped in a clean tea towel before applying to the joint. Sometimes your physiotherapist will show you how to do self-massage for pain relief.

Physiotherapists can also show you how to use a TENS (Transcutaneous Electrical Nerve Stimulation) machine as a way of relieving pain. A TENS machine is a small piece of apparatus that stimulates nerves in the painful area by transmitting a low-level electrical impulse. However, because of the cost of these machines, it may be possible for you to borrow one from your physiotherapist or nurse, to see if the relief provided is worth the cost of purchasing your own TENS machine.

There are many private physiotherapists practising within the community and many of them tend to specialise in different injuries or illnesses. Hence you will get physiotherapists who specialise in back problems and others who may only take clients with sports injuries. There are physiotherapists in the NHS who take general referrals either as in-patients from the hospital wards or as out-patients through a family doctor.

Physiotherapists can advise whether splints, braces or walking aids will be beneficial. If they do not have the relevant items to lend, they can usually give you information on where you will be able to obtain them in the community. Traction may be prescribed. This method of treatment can help where sensations of tingling or numbness are experienced in the arms or legs. Studies suggest it is particularly suitable for people experiencing back pain caused by disc problems. A list of physiotherapists may be found at www.csp.org.uk/physio2u.cfm.

PSYCHOLOGISTS

Psychologists have much to offer a person who is experiencing chronic pain, particularly around the various emotions you may be experiencing as a result of pain. They also have a role to play in providing you with information on and practical assistance for relative treatments for a reduction in pain levels, and also serve to assist you in determining the level of assistance you require. The types of assessments that can be offered include an introduction to a *pain scale* – a personal tool that allows you to keep track of your pain. The scale is between 0–10, with level 10 being the worst pain you can imagine and level 0 being the least pain.

10	**Unbearable Pain**
7–9	**Severe Pain**
4–6	**Moderate Pain**
1–3	**Mild Pain**

Diagram 6: How to rate your pain.

Using this scale, you can assess three levels of pain:
- The pain you are experiencing at the moment
- The worst pain you have ever experienced
- The least pain you have ever experienced

Keeping a pain scale for a month (recording on a daily basis) can provide you with your most frequent level of pain. In conjunction with the pain scale, body awareness is a crucial part of coping with pain. Learning to be aware of your body (e.g. am I hungry, thirsty, tense, hot or cold?) assists you in your observation of pain and the level of pain you are feeling.

Feelings of guilt, worry, anxiety and/or depression result in negative energy and pain compounds easily when your feelings are down. Psychologists can help you work through anxiety, worry or guilt with cognitive behavioural techniques during your session, which you can also take away to put into practice when you are in your own environment. Examples of cognitive behavioural techniques include positive self-talk in which you counteract your negative thoughts and speech with a positive equivalent.

Psychologists can also offer counselling which provides you with the support you may need to get your life back on track. It may be that your self-esteem has taken a battering and the pain you have experienced has left you with less confidence in your abilities. You may have experienced the loss of the lifestyle you had before your pain.

There are a wide range of negative feelings which can often be triggered as a result of loss (e.g. anger and sadness). You may need a period of time to come to terms with these feelings. If you do not deal with these feelings in a reasonable time frame, you may become bogged down in self-pity and depression.

Psychologists can teach you to express your feelings by being open to modes of thought and changes in attitude that might be helpful in improving your life. By learning to express your feelings in a clear, simple, and undemanding way, you can begin to emerge from under the wraps.

Once you realise that you cannot expect others to read your thoughts and you can let others know what pain means or has meant to you without anger or self-pity, you will immediately reduce tensions between you and those close to you – after all, there is an enormous difference between talking and complaining.

Families or carers of people experiencing pain also have their own thoughts and feelings about what is happening in the family because of injury or illness, and psychologists may offer to see individual carers or family groups to work through tensions that may have arisen between family members.

Learning to relax and ease tension and worry is a great reliever of pain. Psychologists can teach you many different ways to relax. You learn the skills in a session with the psychologist, then take those skills away with you to do in your own time in your own environment. Often, some psychologists will use their own relaxation tapes, while others will tell you where you can purchase tapes or compact discs of relaxation music.

In addition, some psychologists will be able to teach you how to use biofeedback yourself. This will give you the ability to control the responses of your body (e.g. anxiety, tenseness), thus allowing you to experience less pain and stress. Biofeedback requires you to be connected to a machine that informs you and the psychologist when you are physically relaxing your body. With sensors placed over specific muscle sites, the psychologist can read the tension in your muscles, the amount of perspiration you are producing, the temperature of your finger and even your heart rate. Using this method the psychologist can tell if you are learning to relax. The goal of this therapy is for you to be able to use this skill when you are facing real stressors away from the psychologist's office.

Research has suggested that biofeedback training can bring about improvement in the number of tender points and morning stiffness in some fibromyalgia patients.

There are psychologists working in the NHS and a number of private psychologists who you can find through the British Psychological Society. If you feel a psychologist would help ease your pain, ask your family doctor to give you a referral to see one.

SOCIAL WORKERS

Social workers can assist you with the practical welfare issues of being unwell (e.g. finances, home help, nursing homes etc.) and also with advice either for yourself or family members.

Finances can change remarkably when there is chronic pain in the family. It may be that a family member has to take some time off work and they may have run out of sick pay entitlements.

Other avenues of financing the family have to be considered and social workers can help to guide you through these options. You can also get advice through the Citizens Advice Bureau and self-help groups (see page 58 for further information). Social workers can help you access the required application forms.

If you are behind in your mortgage or credit payments, and are worried about repossessions, social workers can assist you in contacting your creditors to let them know of your situation and what you would like to do regarding future finances with those organisations. Peace of mind can be achieved by getting your finances sorted out as quickly as you are able to.

Perhaps you are housebound and unable to go out in order to pay accounts, shop or visit your local library. Most social workers have a community resource list of who to contact in these circumstances to assist you.

If you are not in a position to do your housework and there is no one else who can help you, then social services can put you in touch with home helps to assist in this regard. Most communities also have a Meals-on-Wheels service. For a nominal cost they are able to provide a three-course meal from Monday to Friday.

You can contact social workers through your local council. Refer to your local telephone directory for contact details.

WHEELCHAIR SERVICES

The NHS also offers a wheelchair service. You do not have to be totally unable to walk in order to get a chair, but you will need a referral from your therapist or doctor.

Wheelchairs are available in a range of designs and sizes, specifically aimed at meeting different needs. As a consequence, therefore, you will need to be assessed. This may be done in your own home or at the wheelchair centre.

Some people who use wheelchairs can push themselves, while other people need someone to push them. Wheelchairs can be particularly difficult to manoeuvre on uneven ground or on slopes. It is a good idea, if you manage your own chair, to get a strong pair of gloves – good quality golfing gloves are often a favourite. Motorised wheelchairs and scooters are available for some people. Whatever you have it should be serviced regularly and again, your wheelchair centre can arrange to do this for you.

As you can see there is help available, whether it be of a physical and/or psychological nature, or just simple practical assistance, so contact a healthcare professional who will be able to assist you in managing your pain.

CHAPTER FIVE

ALTERNATIVE THERAPIES FOR MANAGING CHRONIC PAIN

This chapter examines some alternative therapies that may help you manage chronic pain – most should be available locally. As discussed in Chapter One (page 10), pain is unique to the person experiencing it; equally the method of pain relief is a matter of individual preference. What suits one person may not suit another. With this in mind, no specific recommendations are given to the types of alternative treatments listed here. It is up to each individual to digest the information provided and consult with a healthcare professional to make a decision as to whether he or she will feel any benefit from the alternative therapies described.

ACUPRESSURE

This is a generic term encompassing a number of massage techniques that use manual pressure to stimulate energy points on the body. Light to medium pressure is applied with the fingers, hands, elbows, knees and feet to the acupuncture points.

Acupressure has its roots in China, and in particular, the philosophy of Taoism. The purpose of an acupressure session is to enhance the body's own recuperative powers by stimulating the body's electromagnetic energy, otherwise known as *chi* in China and *prana* in India. *Chi* is believed to be the motivating life force common to all living things.

An acupressure treatment usually has two or three stages:
- A general energy balancing
- A concentration on the blocked meridians at the root of the imbalance
- A closing technique to seal the energy balancing

Meridians are channels or pathways that carry *chi* and blood through the body – they are not blood vessels. They comprise an invisible network that links together the body's fundamental substances and organs. The meridian system unifies all parts of the body and is essential for the maintenance of harmonious balance. A range of factors can cause blockages in the *chi* network, such as long periods of sitting (e.g. those in sedentary jobs) and internal pressure generated by nervous tension (e.g. stress). Acupressure has had some success in treating back pain, cramps, headaches and migraines. An example of an acupressure technique used to relieve facial aches and pains involves squeezing the web of flesh between the thumb and the index finger for about 5 minutes. The pressure should be towards the index finger. For alleviating nausea, with your wrist facing you, press your thumb on the vein about 5cm down from the wrist for 5–10 minutes.

In the UK acupressure may be offered by acupuncturists and some specialist masseurs.

ACUPUNCTURE

Acupuncture has been widely used in China for approximately 3,000 years and is still practised today. In the West, acupuncture has been adopted as a complementary medicine with many doctors, nurses and physiotherapists learning the skill of inserting fine stainless steel needles into certain points of the body known as meridians.

Research has suggested that acupuncture relieves pain because it causes the release of endorphins. Endorphins are chemicals produced by the pituitary gland, which have a similar effect to that of morphine in changing mood and relieving pain.

Acupuncture is thought to be successful in the management of most muscular pain problems, migraines and toothache. In China it is used as an alternative to anaesthetic in surgical operations. The fact that there are virtually no side-effects from acupuncture can make it an attractive alternative when compared to painkillers and anti-depressant medication.

If, however, you are squeamish about needles, this technique may not be for you, as up to fifteen needles can be inserted into your skin for varying lengths of time. For some pain conditions, you may need to have a course of acupuncture over a period of weeks.

To see any results from acupuncture takes four to six sessions. There is very little pain involved except a slight tingle as the needle pricks the skin. Some people report feeling tired after treatment, so initially it is best to have someone drive you to and from your session until you are aware if any tiredness is affecting you.

All practitioners of acupuncture need to be qualified and to have been trained in anatomy. Before seeking treatment, you need to make sure a practitioner is a member of an acupuncture association and that they use disposable, single-use needles.

ALEXANDER TECHNIQUE

This is a method of re-educating the body and mind to overcome poor habits of posture and movement and to reduce physical and mental tension. Frederick Matthias Alexander, a Tasmanian actor born in 1869, spent nine years studying his own, and other people's, bodily movements to formulate this exercise, which became known as the Alexander Technique.

The method involves lessons during which a qualified practitioner, often using his or her hands, will guide the pupil to experience their innate posture, movement and balance. The focus is on the neck and head and their relationship to the rest of the body. In the initial consultation, the practitioner assesses how you stand, sit, move and breathe.

The Alexander Technique helps to restore your neuromuscular coordination, as old, inhibiting patterns are replaced with freer, more flexible movement. The lessons show people how to use their muscles the way they were originally designed to work. A great deal of practice is involved. The technique is a discipline in which, once the skills are learnt, the pupil can continue on his or her own. The quicker the pupil puts these skills to use, the less need there is to visit a practitioner.

The Alexander Technique can help with back pain, stiff necks, headaches, depressions and for relaxation and economy of movement. It can be a powerful technique for heightening self-awareness and improving overall wellbeing. Initially, the technique can be a little uncomfortable, as you teach your wayward posture to realign itself, but if you persevere you will notice reduced pain levels.

You can find Alexander Technique teachers at some local private clinics and sports centres. A few pain management programmes have a teacher linked to them.

AROMATHERAPY

Research is being conducted into aromas or scents and how they may alter one's moods and thoughts. Aromatherapy involves the use of fragrant oils in massage, baths, oil burners, or burning scented candles. Essential oils are pure oils extracted from the roots, flowers, leaves and stems of plants either through boiling or steaming. The oil can also be extracted by crushing the plants. When using essential oils for massage, the essential oil is diluted with almond oil to make it suitable for the skin.

The scent or fragrance of essential oils is suggested to have a healing power, whether to reduce stress, fight infection, increase energy, relieve headaches or muscular aches and pains. It has been found that these aromas can change brainwave states. Researchers know that when aromatic

Essential oil	Properties	Caution
Geranium	antiseptic, antidepressant anti-inflammatory, balancing, diuretic, refreshing, relaxing skin treatment, warming	
Juniper	aids circulation, analgesic, balancing, antiseptic, cleansing, digestive, soothes nerves, muscle relaxant, refreshing, stimulates appetite, toning	Avoid during pregnancy
Lavender	analgesic, antibacterial, antiseptic, balances emotions, calming, decongestive, digestive, muscle relaxant, refreshing, relaxing, respiratory, sedative, skin treatment, soothing	
Marjoram	antispasmodic, calming, carminative, digestive, muscle relaxant, soothes nerves, respiratory, sedative, warming	Avoid during pregnancy
Patchouli	anti-inflammatory, antiseptic, aphrodisiac, soothes nerves, relaxing, sedative	

molecules drift into the nose, they lock on to receptors there and travel up the olfactory nerves to the brain. One of their destinations is the limbic system, which is where emotions and memory are processed.

Furthermore, essential oils can affect specific areas of the body. Lavender is found to increase alpha-wave activity in the back of the brain, thus bringing about a sense of relaxation. Geranium, juniper and patchouli have been found to relax mood.

Aromatherapists can be found in the local community or you can administer aromatherapy yourself. However, if you decide to opt for the do-it-yourself method, make sure you read the instructions carefully, as a number of essential oils are not suitable for certain medical conditions, such as pregnancy, high blood pressure and epilepsy.

Pharmacies and health food outlets sell the oils, candles and the burners (i.e. the apparatus that the candle fits inside, with the oil being placed in a dish above it).

AUTOGENIC TRAINING

Autogenic training is a technique that originated in Germany and could be thought of as self-hypnosis. Autogenic training consists of repeating certain phrases to yourself in order to relax different parts of your body, for example, repeating the phrase 'my feet are heavy and warm', until you feel your feet become heavy and warm. In conjunction with repeating the phrase, you have to mentally visualise yourself putting your feet into a bowl of warm water. (For more about the techniques of visualisation see Chapter Eight – pages 92–94). Autogenic training has been found to be helpful in treating people with insomnia because of its relaxation effect on all areas of the body. Your psychotherapist may teach it to you.

BOWEN TECHNIQUE

Mr Tom Bowen's system is a unique therapy which involves a series of gentle rolling connective tissue movements using light touch, which realign the body, balance and stimulate the energy flow, empowering the body's own resources to heal itself.

The Bowen Technique stimulates circulation, encourages lymphatic and venous drainage, promotes assimilation of nutrients and elimination of toxins, increases joint mobility and improves posture. Excellent results are reported from those with sporting injuries, backaches and joint discomfort. It is thought that the key to the technique's success is its holistic action.

Many patients report 'feeling' the energy release and flow and a state of deep relaxation during their treatment session. No pain is experienced when undergoing the Bowen Technique. Treatment is ideally performed on low soft tables and moves are effective through clothing. Sessions can last from 10–40 minutes. Relief is often attained after the first session and some clients only need two or three sessions, ideally one week apart. A list of certified practitioners can be obtained from the Bowen Association of the UK.

CHIROPRACTICS

Dr. Daniel David Palmer founded the practice of chiropractics in 1895. The word chiropractic comes from the Greek words *cheiro* and *praktikos* meaning 'done by hand'.

Chiropractors can treat problems that you may be suffering in your bones, joints and muscles, and the effects that these problems can have on the nervous system. They work on all the joints, but particularly focus on the spine. A chiropractor will use their hands to gently manipulate your body. This will improve the efficiency of your nervous system and allow your body's natural healing ability to be released. Chiropractors do not use medicines or drugs and the practice does not involve surgery.

A chiropractic manipulation does not normally feel painful, but you may experience some short-term discomfort, which should quickly pass. You will probably find that later treatments will be more pleasant as your symptoms improve.

Qualified chiropractors can be found in the community in private practice. They are also listed in the telephone directory and at the British Chiropractic Association.

HOMEOPATHY

Homeopathy was discovered by Samuel Hahnemann in the late eighteenth century. Homeopathy comes from the Greek words *homois* and *pathos* meaning 'similar illness' or 'suffering'. Hahnemann's research led him to develop the principle of similars, where he found similar substances could both cure and cause illness.

Homeopathy is very popular among people who prefer natural remedies for their ailments. There are over 2,000 remedies available, each of which have been prepared from plants, herbs, animal products, minerals and chemicals that homeopaths use to treat a variety of illnesses and ailments.

Homeopathy may help some people with chronic pain. You can get further information and advice at the Royal London Homeopathic Hospital in Bloomsbury, London.

HUMOUR THERAPY

Being able to laugh, share a joke or act silly may be hard to envisage when you are in pain; however, laughing and a sense of humour are what pain specialists at the Royal Marsden Oncology Hospital in London have been advocating for their cancer patients for quite some time.

Some pain clinics use humour therapy by getting their patients to lighten up, to have a laugh and not to take life so seriously. People are unique in the topics they find humorous, but there are similarities that people agree on when they describe being humorous (i.e. laughing, feeling good, being relaxed and happy, being accepting and open-minded). Researchers have found that laughter releases endorphins, thus producing a natural high, which makes people happy.

Laughter starts with a smile, so begin the day by looking in the mirror and smiling at yourself. Smile at others – they will not be able to resist smiling back.

Find something that makes you laugh, be it a joke book, audiotape of your favourite comedian or a comedy video. Most of these items can be borrowed from your local library.

HYPNOSIS

Hypnosis produces an induced state of relaxation in which your mind stays narrowly focussed and open to suggestion. No one knows how hypnosis exactly works, but it is thought that it alters the brainwave patterns in the same way as other relaxation techniques. Essentially, the hypnotherapist works with the patient to solve a problem through these relaxation techniques.

The success of hypnosis depends on your willingness to try it. People who do not want to feel out of control often cannot be hypnotised, because they are unable to relax to begin the process. Hypnosis as a form of relaxation is available through some psychologists. There are registered hypnotherapists that just specialise in hypnotism and these are usually found under hypnotherapy in the telephone directory.

It is important to note that hypnosis can be dangerous if administered by an unqualified hypnotist, so make sure that if you choose this type of therapy that the hypnotherapist is properly trained and accredited. People who are suffering from severe mental disorders are best advised to avoid hypnosis.

MASSAGE

Massage is probably one of the oldest therapies known if we look at ancient Greek and Roman histories. Massage is used to relax the body and mind and is said to improve circulation, high blood pressure, headaches, aching backs and necks. Massage is not suitable for people who are suffering from varicose veins, phlebitis (vein inflammation), thrombosis (blood clotting) or simply during an acute flare-up of pain.

The touch used in massage can vary from stroking and applying pressure to kneading and drumming. A massage session can last 20–40 minutes depending on what the massage therapist assesses you will find beneficial to your condition and may involve the use of aromatherapy oils. Before the session begins, you will be asked to strip down to your underwear and lie on the massage table.

At the end of your massage, you should feel relaxed in both mind and body. You can either visit a qualified masseur or massage your own body parts (be sure to get advice from a professional before you do this).

MEDITATION

It is in Eastern philosophy that we find the origin of meditation where Buddhist monks and the Yogis of India have been practising meditation for centuries. The word meditation comes from the Latin word *meditari*, which means 'frequently'. It is essential to practise meditation frequently in order to feel its positive effects. Meditation has three different avenues:

- As a means of problem solving (known as insight meditation)
- As a means of achieving what we set our mind to (known as creative meditation)
- To relax our bodies and minds (known as health meditation)

It is the last avenue that people in Western societies tend to use as a means of reducing their stress levels.

Zen Buddhism refers to meditation as just sitting and doing nothing which, when the process of meditation is learned, is correct. However, it is not that simple, initially. You have to be in a mode of single-minded concentration, blocking out all intrusions on the mind to create a state of being rather than letting the mind wander to a state of doing.

Meditation needs to be performed frequently for the techniques to be learned. It is recommended that people practise meditation once, preferably twice, a day. People with pain and insomnia can benefit from meditation. Please note that it is dangerous to meditate while driving or operating machinery. More information on the process of meditation can be found in Chapter Eight (see pages 96–98).

MUSIC THERAPY

Music therapy is a non-pharmacological approach to reducing fear, anxiety, stress or grief in chronically ill patients. It is just beginning to make a mark in the UK as a method of treating pain and associated stress, yet many are already reporting it to be the best way to lower stress. Some researchers have found that in studies with chronic pain patients, the use of music can cause patients to have a higher tolerance of pain.

Music therapy may sound too easy to work, but many of the sensations arising from music and pain are processed in the same areas of the brain. These areas also coordinate our emotional responses. It is believed that by focussing on or responding to music, we can block or distract the body's response to pain. With this form of relaxation, we can decrease muscle tension and increase endorphin levels. While the level of pain does not change, having less tension and anxiety can make the pain more tolerable.

For maximum results, it is helpful to try music therapy in combination with deep abdominal breathing or deep muscle relaxation – this will enhance the feeling of inner peace. (Breathing and deep muscle relaxation are discussed further in Chapter Eight – see pages 89–99).

When undergoing music therapy, you may like to choose music that is slightly slower than your heart rate or approximately 60 beats per minute – this rhythm encourages your heart to slow down. Listen to music at a comfortable volume. If discomfort increases, try increasing the volume and decrease the volume as the discomfort decreases. It is helpful to have earphones or a headset, as then you'll avoid disturbing others. Mark time to the music – tap out the rhythm with your finger on the chair arm or tap your feet on the floor. This helps you concentrate on the music rather than your pain.

Music therapy is not physically or mentally demanding and can be used up to one hour per session. Of course having music you find enjoyable to listen to makes all the difference. There are some beautiful relaxation music tapes and compact discs in your local music store – from the sound of trickling rainforest pools to the lapping movements of waves at the seashore – or you may prefer something more up-beat that lends itself to feet and finger tapping.

OSTEOPATHY

Osteopathy was founded by Dr Andrew Taylor Still in the nineteenth century. Osteopathy involves the use of manipulation, physical therapy and postural education – the latter two being the difference between osteopaths and chiropractors.

Osteopaths have a belief that all our vital organs are controlled by spinal nerves and that injuries which involve the musculoskeletal system may aggravate already diseased or stressed internal organs.

During an initial assessment, an osteopath will carefully observe the contours of the body, noting any distortions in spinal alignment and posture. Working from head to toe, the osteopath will ask you to make certain movements in order to assess both your flexibility and range of movement. He or she will then palpate the body by laying hands on the skin to assess the condition of the skin, the underlying tissues and organs.

The osteopath will need to have records of your medical history and details about the onset of the condition that you wish him or her to treat. From this assessment the osteopath will devise a treatment plan that should be beneficial to you.

The majority of osteopaths work on patients who have back and neck problems, or sports injuries. Osteopaths are registered in the UK and some have medical training.

Treatment sessions are usually 20–30 minutes long and pain may be experienced during and after treatment, but this will usually disappear within the space of 1–2 days.

QI GONG

Qi Gong (pronounced Chi Goong) originates from China and has a history spanning 3,000 years. Qi Gong can be performed while standing, sitting or lying down, using special breathing techniques where the pupil learns to focus his or her mind.

There is another type of Qi Gong that is mobile rather than stationary. The latter employs movements and massage while maintaining balance between the mind and emotion. All the joints and parts of the body are moved slowly and gently in order to convey Qi through the meridians, thereby generating the Qi energy properly. Internally, Qi Gong enhances the spirit, the Qi and the mind while externally it strengthens the body (i.e. the bones and tendons).

Qi Gong exercise can regulate the functioning of the brain and promote the functioning of the circulatory, digestive and other systems. Qi Gong diligently practised acts as a preventative health measure as the body will be strengthened and more resistant to disease. No pain is felt from these gentle movements. How often you practise Qi Gong depends on factors such as your age and your medical condition. It is suggested that those new to Qi Gong start off with two 10-minute sessions and work up to 20- and then 40-minute sessions twice a day. As you work through the process you will notice a general feeling of well-being in your body and mind.

Sometimes it is difficult to find teachers of Qi Gong, particularly in rural areas. However, if you wish to try this form of therapy you can contact your local Citizens Advice Bureau, or do some research on the internet. Once you are able to find a teacher you will most likely find that their qualifications come from studying under the masters of this gentle art.

REFLEXOLOGY

Reflexology originated in China some 5,000 years ago and involves stroking or applying pressure to one part of the body in order to effect changes in another part. Its aim is to stimulate the body's own natural ability to heal itself. For example, the feet are known as the mirror of the body to reflexologists. The left and right feet correspond to the left and right sides of the body and the soles of the feet connect in some way to the organs. By massaging the feet, the body loosens tensions or blockages that stop life energy from circulating freely in the body. Free flowing energy helps the body regain its natural balance, harmony and health.

Reflexology stimulates blood circulation to nourish the body and stimulates the lymph system. It is particularly recommended for conditions such as headaches, migraines and stress. Two or three treatments usually offer some improvement. Reflexology is not suitable for people suffering from arthritis in their feet, diabetes, osteoporosis or phlebitis. Treatment should be by a qualified practitioner and you can get details at www.aor.org.uk.

REIKI

Reiki is an energy healing system based on ancient Tibetan knowledge, rediscovered by the Japanese theologian, Dr Mikao Usui. During reiki sessions, universal life energy is channelled to clients. Reiki practitioners transmit this energy by gently placing their hands in specific positions on the client's body without exerting pressure, while following the body's shape. Heat will be felt by the reiki practitioner to indicate the source of the problem.

The purpose of reiki is to supply the body with additional energy and those who have experienced reiki have noticed the physical and emotional benefits of this type of therapy. Reiki can be a relaxing meditative experience.

Reiki practitioners have been trained under certified masters of the art at their own expense. There are three levels of competency the student must reach before being able to practise:

- Level 1: traditional hand movements
- Level 2: level 1 plus healing at a distance
- Level 3: level 2 plus the master symbol

Reiki sessions usually run for one hour in which the practitioner links the client to cosmic, radiant energy, opens chakras (i.e. channels), or attunes that individual, as a receiver, to universal life.

Reiki has been found to be particularly beneficial in the elderly, for arthritis or osteoporosis, as it may help relieve a person's pain and improve their mobility.

SHIATSU

Shiatsu has been described as acupuncture without needles or a technique similar to acupressure.

Shiatsu is Japanese for finger pressure, but the knees, knuckles, palms and feet may also be used. Shiatsu originated in Japan some 1,500 years ago. The Shiatsu techniques are called *do-in* and *tsubo*. Both techniques create a state of deep relaxation and are used for managing chronic pain and other difficult medical problems. Each Shiatsu session covers the whole body and includes pressing with the knee or elbow to stimulate blood flow and stretching and squeezing to unblock energy.

Shiatsu treatment is firm and robust, even described by some as 'invigorating', so it is not suitable for pregnant women or those with high blood pressure, epilepsy, arthritis, osteoporosis, thrombosis, varicose veins or the elderly infirm.

Shiatsu is mainly used to treat existing conditions, their symptoms and the source of these problems, including anxiety, back pain, headache, migraine and stress. Shiatsu should always be performed by a qualified professional and details can be found in local telephone directories under Alternative or Complementary Medicines and Therapies.

SELF-HELP GROUPS

There are a number of disease- and pain-related self-help groups which you may access via the Pain Society website, which can be found at www.painsociety.org or through your local Yellow Pages. Self-help groups offer information, education and support. Some also raise funds for and/or commission research.

The NHS Self-Management Programme, developed by Pete Moore and David Matthews, has been designed to encourage and enable people with chronic pain to take more control. For further information see the Addresses section (page 102).

TAI CHI

Tai Chi is a slow, graceful exercise that gently tones the body, both inside and out. It may have the following benefits: lowering blood pressure, improving circulation, and relaxation. It has also been approved by back specialists. Practising Tai Chi on a regular basis builds up muscles, energy, balance and coordination while calming the mind through breathing and meditation. Tai Chi Chuan, meaning 'supreme ultimate power', is one of the gentler forms of Tai Chi and offers an effective way to relieve stress, tone the body and improve general health.

Learning the form (i.e. movement) within Tai Chi can be a very challenging process – especially at first – because we must teach our bodies to move in a slightly different manner. The movements are slow and can take up to 20–35 minutes on average to work through. Many Tai Chi teachers teach the form in three phases. When learning the movements, each phase is practised until correct and then they are all joined together to create one continuous movement. The mind is calm, the body is relaxed and the head and shoulders hang loose, never rising. The spine is straight and both the head and body move as one. The knees are directly over the toes, as in a simple lunge. The weight moves from one leg to the other, creating a fluidity of movement. The whole body is gently exercised and toned by these movements and when done correctly, the body's energy flow (*chi*) is increased, circulating around and invigorating every part of the body.

You will be able to find details at your local library or in the telephone directory.

YOGA

Yoga originated in India and dates back almost 5,000 years. Hatha yoga is a combination of physical poses, known as *asanas*, interspersed with breathing techniques, known as *pranayama*. Yoga can also involve meditation as a means of enhancing clarity of thought and inner strength. (Breathing and meditation are discussed further in Chapter Eight – see pages 89–91 and 96–98.)

Hatha yoga is particularly beneficial for people who are reluctant to exercise because it is taught in stages – beginner's, intermediate and advanced. If you suffer chronic pain you should try a beginner's or an over-50s yoga class because these are the classes that progress slowly, encouraging you to do what you can, rather than expecting you to do the same as everyone else.

Breathing or breath is very important in yoga, as it not only gives the body oxygen but also energy, known as *chi*. Movements in the body affect our breathing: for example, when we start to run our breathing quickens, when we lie down our breathing slows. Breathing in yoga is slow and rhythmic.

There are many ways of doing yoga poses. Some are gentle, some are strengthening and some are strenuous. The type of yoga exercises needed for people in chronic pain are gentle so that they assist in relieving stress and revitalising and healing the body.

Yoga is offered as day and evening classes in many areas. When inquiring about yoga, ask the teacher as to the type of class taught. Usually yoga of a beginner's or over-50s level is of a gentler nature. There are many good books in the local library and even videos that teach yoga. However, you will probably find it more beneficial if you attend a class initially and learn the correct breathing techniques and become familiar with the poses.

Yoga is pleasant and enjoyable, and when you discover that yoga does indeed improve your overall health, you will want to find time for it in your daily schedule.

It is important to note that if you are pregnant, you should only practise a gentle form of yoga that contains safe poses for pregnant women. You should also let your teacher know of any underlying or recent illness.

Access to all the therapies described in this chapter may be found through information provided by your local library, evening class lists, Yellow Pages (see "Alternative or Complementary Medicines or Therapies") or via the internet.

CHAPTER SIX

PHYSICAL SELF-HELP

Body awareness teaches a person with chronic pain to have respect for pain by balancing activity and rest. This is called pacing. You will accomplish more if you rest frequently, rather than continuing to push to the point of collapse. Your body will replenish its energy supply much more quickly if you take short breaks between tasks. Short breaks are much better than long breaks because long breaks tend to place you in one position for too long (i.e. sitting in front of the television engrossed in a programme or lying on the bed and falling asleep). This may cause stiffness or soreness when commencing with your tasks again.

Pain can be nature's warning that too much work has been done for too long, usually in an awkward posture. If this is you, it is time to make some changes in your life by adopting the following perspectives.

1. Learning to accept assistance from others

This can be hard if you are used to doing everything yourself to your own standards. You will have to learn to accept different standards of work and be grateful that you have received an offer of help. You will have to get over any feelings of frustration or failure in that you are no longer able to do some of the things you could do before your injury or illness. You may also have to overcome your pride and ask others for their assistance.

2. Learning to leave tasks unfinished

Learning to leave tasks unfinished may be difficult if you're a perfectionist, but once you are able to do this, you are acknowledging that you can balance work with rest periods, rather than trying to complete the task and be out of action for a couple of days because you have overdone it. Remember that quality of life is important. Quality may be friends and family who visit to spend time with you, not to see how clean your house is.

3. Learning to use equipment and devices that expand the quality of your life

There are many labour-saving devices on the market that reduce the time and energy needed to complete everyday tasks. For example, an upright vacuum cleaner may be easier to use than a barrel cleaner that involves lots of bending. Owning lighter chairs that are easier to lift or move when you are vacuuming or mopping is also beneficial. Placing a basket at the top and bottom of the staircase for transferring items from upstairs to downstairs and vice versa, will conserve your energy.

You can also conserve your energy by planning ahead what you have to do, by eliminating unnecessary tasks, by sitting to do some of your chores (e.g. ironing or meal preparation) and by alternating light and heavy tasks. Planning allows you to pace yourself evenly throughout the week, which is very important in overcoming the effects of pain while doing activities. Research has found that many people with pain get into a cycle of over-extending themselves when they are having a good day, thereby exacerbating their pain and having to rest for the next couple of days until the pain eases. They then do too much again, to catch up with what they need to do. Planning allows you to be organised and get the work done with rest breaks and daily exercise in between.

To plan effectively, obtain a diary and start to look at your week. What do you want to achieve this week? Do you have to do everything or can you delegate some of the jobs you cannot do to other people? Try to sort out the jobs into daily (e.g. washing dishes), weekly (e.g. vacuuming) and monthly (e.g. washing the car) categories. As you put these tasks into your diary, remember to allow time to rest and don't cram all the heavy jobs together; mix them with lighter tasks. For example, make the bed followed by writing a letter to a friend or relative (or a similar restful activity). Dust one room then listen to the radio or some music. Vacuum the room you have dusted, then eat a meal and take a relaxation break, perhaps do your daily exercise (maybe a short walk to the shops to pick up things you may need for the evening meal). Try to plan tasks for the time of day or week when you are feeling your best. Someone with arthritis may have difficulty making their bed first thing in the morning and may find it better to have the first task of the day washing the breakfast dishes. Someone waking with a headache may find it easier to go for his or her walk after breakfast, to practise relaxation and get some fresh air to lessen the pain of the headache.

EXERCISE

Unfortunately, household tasks do not count as daily exercise. It is a well-known fact that people in pain will tell you the last thing they want to do is exercise. However, pain management programmes incorporate daily exercise into their programmes, not only to mobilise stiff joints but also to motivate you to take responsibility for managing your pain. Exercise is part of the overall management plan for someone with chronic pain. Exercising correctly will not only improve your quality of life but will assist you in maintaining your overall general health. The benefits of exercise include:

- Maintaining increased movement
- Improved muscle tone
- Improved circulation
- Improved joint stability
- Relief from stiffness, pain and tension

- Help in promoting sleep
- Help in preventing osteoporosis
- Weight control

Many painful physical conditions are a result of negative lifestyle habits that have been accumulated over a lifetime. For example, working in sedentary positions; not taking enough exercise; poor posture; lifting heavy items the wrong way; obesity that puts extra strain on joints; poor diets and excess alcohol and cigarettes.

However, while we may be paying for negative lifestyle habits, it is never too late to change and start putting something positive back into our lives. The key to managing pain through exercise is to make a commitment and allow time for it in your daily programme.

Next time you visit your family doctor or healthcare practitioner, discuss with him or her the exercises you used to do, those you would like to do, and the programme you are planning to adopt. Do not overdo exercising, particularly in the beginning; instead, start by trying the movements slowly and carefully. Don't be alarmed if an exercise causes mild discomfort which lasts for a few minutes; after all, if you've not exercised for some time your muscles will be a little stiff and sore. However, do stop exercises that aggravate pre-existing pain. That is, do not force movement past the point of pain, and seek advice.

POSTURE

The following information involves body awareness to correct negative posture habits.

Bending

Long-handled sticks with prongs on the end can be bought to save bending down to pick up dropped items. Long-handled barbecue tongs do the job just as well. If you have neither of these gadgets, then look at what you have nearby on which to place your hands for support while you squat down to pick an item up. Including squats in your exercise programme can also make it easier to bend.

Sitting

Use a firm chair with good support to help you assume the best posture when sitting. Do not slouch. Support the entire length of your spine against the back of the chair and keep your knees level with your hips by using a footstool or pouffe.

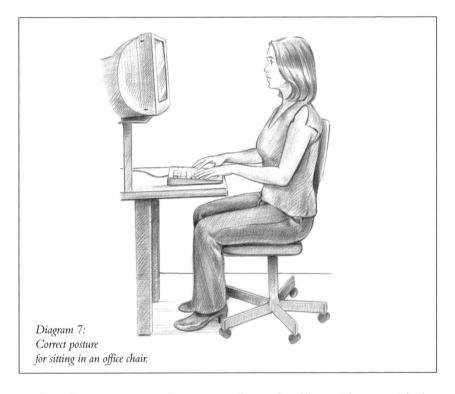

Diagram 7:
Correct posture
for sitting in an office chair.

If you have to sit at work, your employer should provide you with the equipment you need. Otherwise, on upright chairs, use a back roll (or roll up a towel) to give more support to the centre or bottom of your back. Make sure your feet are placed together on the floor. If your feet will not reach the floor, use a foot rest or build a stack of telephone directories on which to place your feet. When seated, the table or desk should be at elbow height (see Diagram 7).

To get up from a low chair, put your feet on the floor first, then lean forward and shift your body weight over your feet and stand up by straightening your knees. Try to avoid easy chairs and sofas that you sink into as they give very little, if any, support. Get up and move every 20–30 minutes. Do not cross your legs, as this stretches the sciatic nerve and back muscles and is not good for circulation in the legs.

Some of the modern ideas to improve sitting postures include the ergonomic chair that has no back but separate pads to support the knees, or the exercise ball where, because there is no back support, the back must be kept straight to maintain balance. Perching stools may also be useful. They let you sit in situations where you would normally stand, such as to iron or cook. All this equipment can be sought through your therapists.

Sleeping

Use a firm mattress. If your mattress is not firm and you are not in the market for a new one, an alternative is to try placing a piece of board between the mattress and the bed base. If you are experiencing acute back pains, sleep with a pillow or blanket rolled under your knees and a neck pillow under your head.

An orthopaedic specialist may advise you to put two or three pillows under your knees and have no pillows under your head, thereby taking some of the pressure off your spine. This suggestion is in conflict with some rheumatologists who believe that flexing or bending the knees for long periods of time may eventually lead to deformity and certainly pain when straightening them to get out of bed. The latter two statements offer conflicting advice so if in doubt as to what you should do, you can either discuss it with your family doctor or try out the position yourself for observation and experience of whether there is pain relief or not.

Fatigue is often an insidious companion to pain and you will need to heed your own body's warning signals (e.g. body aching, increased pain, insomnia). Allow yourself to rest completely, even if it is only for a short time. Avoid caffeine and spicy foods prior to bedtime. Do not take your worries to bed with you, as your mind and body need to be relaxed. (Worry is discussed further in Chapter Seven – see pages 83–88.) Avoid stimulating activities such as exercise or reading, as these involve the mind and body and make it hard to settle. Unwind slowly before going to bed by trying some relaxation techniques (see Chapter Eight – pages 89–99) or listening to some relaxing music.

When lying on your side keep your knees and hips bent. If there is pain in one leg, lie on the opposite side and support the painful leg with a pillow between the knees. When rising from lying down, roll onto one side, slide your legs over the edge of the bed as you push up from the side. Do not attempt to sit up straight from a lying position.

Driving

When driving or riding in a car, stop for a break when you need to. Get out of the car and walk around and try a few stretches. When driving, sit close to the steering wheel by adjusting the car seat. There are various car seats and cushions that you can purchase to give you extra support and comfort. To get into the car, sit on the seat first and then rotate both feet into the car. To get out of the car, do the reverse, rotate your feet out onto the ground and then stand up.

Pulling and pushing

Activities such as vacuuming, mowing the lawn or walking with a buggy all involve pulling and pushing movements. Use the power position when undertaking these activities. Lean forward from the ankles, brace your feet firmly and push against the ground. Ensure your body is in correct alignment with the object to avoid twisting and strain. When you are using a vacuum cleaner, put one foot forward and shift your body weight from one leg to the other as you push the vacuum. Every so often change the foot that is forward and switch the hand that pushes the vacuum.

It is always better to push than to pull an object. If you have to pull an object, place one foot under or past the object, and one foot in the direction you are pulling. Shift your body weight from your front leg to your back leg when pulling.

Safe lifting and lowering

When lifting or lowering an object, bring the load as close to you as possible. Hug the load. Avoid any twisting or bending of the spine as you lift or lower a load. Lead into a turn with your feet and try to keep movements smooth and controlled. Always bend the knees rather than the back. The trick to being comfortable in any of the latter postural activities is to avoid staying in one position for too long.

SELF CARE

Sometimes when in pain or suffering depression, it is easy to let the care of your personal self slip. It's too much bother to put on fresh clothes every day, a struggle to do up buttons or bend down to tie shoelaces. The water from the shower makes your body feel bruised and drying yourself is such an effort. However, looking after your personal care doesn't need to be too difficult. Here are some helpful hints.

Dressing

Clothing can be restrictive to people who have limited movement and dressing can take longer and expend a lot of energy to the point of exhaustion for some.

Make sure you always allow yourself time to dress so you don't have to rush, and can be seated while doing it. If possible, have a footstool nearby to save bending when putting on shoes, socks or tights. Pharmacies and independent living centres have many gadgets to make the task of dressing much easier, including long-handled shoehorns in plastic or metal for putting on shoes, aids for putting on socks or stockings, dressing sticks for pulling clothing over shoulders and loopers for fastening buttons. Clothing that has fastenings at the front is much easier to fasten. A loop or ring on a zip makes it much easier to pull up or down.

If you are a small woman (who does not have thoracic spine pain), you can get away with wearing a sports bra that has no fastenings – just pull it over your head. However, for those who need more support, or who have shoulder pain, wear a front-fastening bra – which is easier to do up. If you still have plenty of use in the bras you already possess, turn the bra to the front to fasten, then turn it to the back and slip your arms into the straps and pull them over your shoulders.

Night attire made of satin material makes for ease of movement in bed.

Wearing shoes or trainers with Velcro fastening eliminates tying shoelaces, but if you prefer lace-ups, you can purchase elastic shoelaces in the popular colours of brown, black and white. Elastic shoelaces allow for more flexibility when fastening shoes. For those with arthritis, some people have found that sheepskin slippers help to reduce the pain as sheepskin keeps the joints warm. You can even purchase sheepskin mittens. When buying shoes, buy the best you can afford. Make sure they are comfortable with low or flat heels and preferably with padded inner soles, as these can be removed to allow more room should your feet get swollen. The best uppers are made of soft but not spongy leather. Leather soles are alright for standing or walking short distances, however for exercise or serious walking, look for rubber soles that provide maximum shock absorbing capabilities.

Always try on shoes later in the day, when your feet are at their most swollen. If you do not have the right pair of shoes in your wardrobe, then seriously consider purchasing a pair because the right shoes can make all the difference to pain in the lower back, hips, legs and knees.

A watch that has a stretch band may be easier to put on than one with a strap and buckle that needs fastening.

If you like to accessorise your clothing with jewellery, then try beads or a chain that goes over your head, rather than those that have fiddly hooks and eyes.

Showering

Showering is generally easier than bathing and a walk-in shower with adequate room for a plastic chair is desirable. A bath can be helpful if you get pain relief from soaking in heated water. There are also some spas you can buy that fit into the bath that is already in your bathroom. Use a non-skid mat on the floor of the bathroom and a non-slip suction mat in the shower or bath. Grip rails on the side of the bath or the walls of the shower give firm support when getting up from a sitting position. If you are unable to get into a bath, a bath board you can sit on may be helpful, as when you lift your feet into the bath, you don't run the risk of slipping. Bath boards can be purchased from independent living centres and pharmacies, or see your occupational therapist who may be able to get hold of these for you.

Soap-on-a-rope saves bending if you drop the soap – just hang it on your shower or bath taps. Another idea to save you dropping the soap is to cut the leg off a pair of tights, drop the soap in and tie it to the shower taps, making it easy to reach at chest height. A hand-held showerhead can make a lot of difference, as it allows you to direct the water to any part of your body and away from you, should the water temperature fluctuate. Most plumbers can install these or you can purchase a rubber one that fits onto the taps on the bath from large supermarkets or hardware stores.

Drying oneself can become a chore if you become hot and flustered while trying to complete this task. A simple way is to have a towelling robe to slip into or a chair with a towel draped over it while you sit and dry yourself with another towel. Have your clothing to put on nearby.

Cleaning your teeth

When cleaning your teeth, sit if you need to, and rest your elbows on the hand basin to give you some support. Have all the things you need close together. If the toothpaste in the tube is hard to squeeze, try a push top dispenser or one of the gadgets available through your pharmacist. If you cannot manage to clean your teeth as much as you would like, don't forget that you can use an electric toothbrush. Its efficient, rotating action helps to eliminate the wrist movement required for brushing teeth with a manual toothbrush.

Shaving and hair care

Shaving with an electric razor is quicker than a manual shave. If you prefer a manual shave, sit down and rest your elbows on the basin for support and to prevent aching arms. If you find it difficult to hold a hairdryer, see if you can buy a lightweight one at the chemist. Long-handled combs and brushes are available for hair care. There are barbers and hairdressers who will visit you in your home to wash, cut, colour or perm your hair. You can usually find them listed in the telephone directory, or an advertisement on the community noticeboard or local newspapers.

Toileting

Handrails by the toilet will make it easier for getting up and down. You can also purchase raised toilet seats from pharmacies and independent living centres that clip on to the original toilet seat, or there are toilet seats that are raised to fit over the original toilet.

People with chronic pain often get constipated because of reduced exercise and the effect of some medications. Drinking plenty of water to soften the stools and making sure there is roughage in your diet can help when opening your bowels.

Regular exercise also helps bowel movements. Rushing through toileting and being stressed can add to constipation. Sit down and take your time!

SEXUAL ACTIVITY

Sexual problems as a result of pain are very common. Sexual problems in relation to pain usually occur for the following reasons:
- Loss of sexual desire or function due to medication
- Loss of sexual desire or function due to illness
- Diminished sense of personal attractiveness due to pain/disability
- Increase in pain during lovemaking because of certain movements or positions

The fear of hurting yourself may be distracting and can interfere with your responses. If it is painful, you may want to use the diagrams in this section to start a discussion with your partner about the different positions you could use.

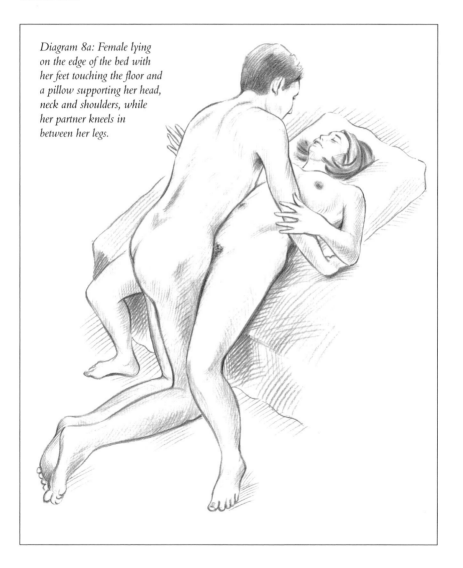

Diagram 8a: Female lying on the edge of the bed with her feet touching the floor and a pillow supporting her head, neck and shoulders, while her partner kneels in between her legs.

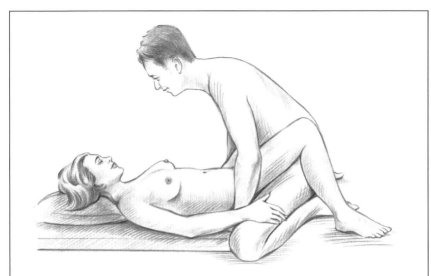

Diagram 8b: Female lying with legs raised while her partner kneels in between her legs.

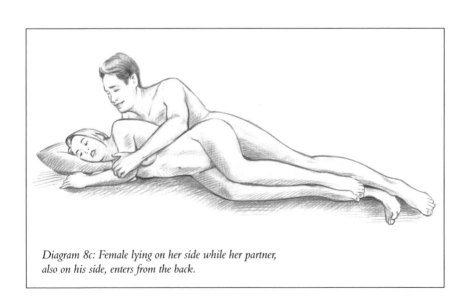

Diagram 8c: Female lying on her side while her partner,
also on his side, enters from the back.

What is needed to address most of these sexual problems is communication and understanding. It also helps to have a good sense of humour.

Remember that intimacy with your partner does not always have to be sexual intercourse. For example, intimacy can be through touch, exploring one another's body by stroking, touching, kissing, cuddling or massaging. Oral sex may be an alternative. Vibrators can also provide pleasure without any physical exertion. Your local library may stock some helpful books.

HOUSEHOLD TASKS

When suffering from chronic pain, it is often difficult to complete domestic chores. Here are a few tips on making these jobs less painful.

Bed making

A higher bed means less bending. If your bed is not high enough, maybe someone in the family can raise the bed up on blocks for you. Make sure the bed is pulled out from the wall so that you can get around both sides of it. If the bed has to be up against a wall for space purposes, putting castors on its base will make it easier to pull out when bed making and pushing back when finished. One trip around the bed should be all that is necessary. Move down one side of the bed, smoothing and tucking, then up the other side, instead of running backwards and forwards.

Try to arrange washing the bedroom linen when your partner or someone else in the family is home to help you. When changing sheets, if you have a bedspread or blankets, roll them down to the foot of the bed and drape them over a chair. Fold them back after the sheets have been replaced. Have cleaned sheets folded in such a way that they can be put in the middle of the bed. Unfold towards the head and tuck in then unfold towards the foot and tuck in.

To eliminate frequent walking backwards and forwards learn to make each corner completely – tuck in the sheets and blankets at the same time before moving to the next one. Fitted sheets and duvets make bed making much easier. Always have someone else turn the mattress for you – ask another family member, friend or neighbour.

Dusting

If buying new furniture, you may wish to think about choosing furniture with a simple shape, which is light in colour, as dust does not collect as quickly on this type of furniture. Use a long-handled feather duster for out of reach places. Sit on a stool for lower areas to save bending. Ornaments are dust collectors, so if you have to have them put them into a cupboard with glass doors. This way you can admire them without accumulated dust.

Vacuuming, sweeping and mopping

As mentioned previously, an upright vacuum cleaner may be easier for you to use, however, if you own a barrel vacuum cleaner make sure it has handles long enough to save bending. Invest in a turbo-head for your vacuum cleaner, as this power suction tends to remove the hard work of vacuuming. Do not attempt the whole house in one day; instead, concentrate on one room at a time. When using a broom, sweep in long strokes, pushing the broom wherever possible. Avoid twisting the body. Use a long-handled hand brush and dustpan to remove any dirt. Squeeze mops are light and effective. A plastic bucket is lighter than a metal one. Put the bucket on a platform with castors. You can either make one or purchase one used for moving pot plants around.

Bathroom

Have cleaning equipment on hand (e.g. in the vanity unit cupboard). Clean as you use and encourage family members to do the same. Some of the newer cleaners are ideal and take away the hard labour as you just spray and then rinse off some 10–15 minutes later. An extractor fan in the bathroom does not allow mould and mildew to build up.

Oven

Cook in oven bags – they certainly save a lot of the splattering of fat and grease on the oven interior when cooking. Wipe out the oven while it's still warm, as this cuts down on cleaning. When you have to clean thoroughly use an oven cleaning spray. Take out the shelves and soak them in hot soapy water, which will soften spills and grease. Wipe the shelves and trays with a damp cloth and the interior of the oven with hot soapy water and then replace the shelves.

Hotplates

Try to mop up spills as you go and wipe the surface with a warm, soapy, damp cloth. When cleaning ceramic oven tops, use a ceramic oven top cleaner. Hotplates are easy to keep clean when buffed with a paper towel and cleaner.

Food preparation

Sit on a stool with back support or a perching stool when at the kitchen worktop preparing food or sit on a chair at the kitchen table. Plan the meal and organise the equipment and ingredients you need prior to starting preparation. Make sure all the kitchen equipment is lightweight. Store the equipment in easy-to-pull-out drawers rather than kitchen cupboards that require you to kneel down to see what is on the bottom shelf at the back of the cupboard. Hang up any kitchen equipment you use regularly (e.g. carving knives, vegetable peeler, fish slicer etc.).

Slide saucepans on the stove, rather than lift, where possible. Invest in an electric tin opener and gadgets to help you open jars and bottles. Add a piece of string or large ring to your sink plug to make emptying the sink easier. Elbow taps on the kitchen sink are easier to handle than the ones you turn. However if you have older style taps, there is a gadget called a tap turner that you can purchase, or get from your occupational therapist.

Cook one-dish meals, such as casseroles, as these are easier to prepare, cook and serve. Make extra and freeze, to be reheated at a later time. Ready-prepared meals from the supermarket are a good alternative from time to time. If you find peeling vegetables difficult, buy the frozen variety, as there is now a large choice available. Buy potatoes that are already washed and cook them in their jackets. Use a non-slip board for carving meat or grating cheese. You can buy non-slip rubber mats from the chemist to go under chopping boards, plates etc.

Laundry

Sort laundry on a bench to save bending. Use a spray or soaker to remove stains, which saves scrubbing. If your washing machine is low, have it raised on blocks. When your washing is finished, have a laundry trolley ready to place the clothes in and push to the washing line if you have one. A washing trolley is a good investment as it saves bending to hang the clothes on the clothesline. Have pegs in a container in the laundry trolley. Repeat the same process when clothes are dry. Replace pegs in the container and fold the washing for ironing from the clothes-line.

Look for a lightweight iron, as some irons are quite heavy and cumbersome to use. If you have the space, leave your ironing board set up. Do not do unnecessary ironing (e.g. sheets and underwear). Get used to sitting when ironing. The ironing board should be 5cm (2 inches) above your thighs and your feet should touch the floor. If you would rather stand to iron, have a footrest upon which to place one foot and change feet regularly, or try a perching stool. Make sure your ironing basket is in easy reach so you don't have to bend and twist your body to get the clothes on to the ironing board. Have coat hangers ready on a rail to use for freshly ironed garments.

Shopping

Shopping can be an unpleasant task if you are in pain and you shop at popular times (e.g. late night shopping and Saturday mornings), or you are stressed and have not got a list of what you need. A memo board placed on the fridge is a good idea because as you run out of items, you or your family members can place them on the memo board. Try to shop during off peak hours. Think about pacing your shopping. You may like to do a little every day or, if you have help, go for one-stop shopping, where you do not have to run all over town to pick things up from different places. Opt for a shallow shopping trolley with good wheels and push in an upright position. When in the checkout queue, rest your foot on the trolley rung, alternating your feet. Choose shops that have seats for rest periods. Try to use the same supermarket, that way you get to know where items you need are placed and it cuts down on the time factor of shopping. If possible, avoid taking small children shopping with you as shopping is tiring enough. Consider shops that will deliver your goods if getting them into the car is a problem, or ask the shop for some assistance to take the goods back to your car. Try to avoid the plastic carry bags as they put extra strain on your fingers. You will be caring for the environment as well as your health if you use your own bag or a shopping trolley. There are also numerous websites that sell groceries online. The benefit is that you don't have to face the supermarket to get your groceries and you can arrange a delivery time for your goods that suits you.

When you are paying household accounts, think of the easiest way for you to do it. This may be by post, direct debit, telephone or online. Alternatively, you may decide to go out to pay them in person, as part of your exercise programme.

Gardening

Have a low maintenance garden for less effort. Consider paving and raised garden beds. Courtyard gardens are presently the trend. Use long-handled garden tools, neatly stored so that you can place your hands on what is needed without difficulty. If mowing, push rather than pull, using a lightweight mower. If your house is large, mow in sections and rest in between.

Mulch garden beds to keep weeds down. If you have to weed, use a 'kneeler' with handles to help you get up and down. A 'kneeler' has a padded area to rest your knees. Do not stay in this position for too long – set yourself a time limit. What does not get done in one day can be done in another. Better still, why not purchase a commercial weed killer that fits onto your garden hose and weed by this means. When using a spade to dig out compost, position yourself by flexing your knees and be close to the compost pile. Limit the load amount and use a light-weight wheelbarrow to transfer to garden beds.

Avoid lifting heavy plant pots. Before transplanting plants into heavy pots, place the pot on to a platform with castors so it is easy to move it to where you want the plant to stand.

Use lightweight plastic garden furniture, so you can move it where you wish. Plastic furniture is easily cleaned with the garden hose.

EMPLOYMENT

There are a number of issues to be considered if you suffer from chronic pain. The major issue would have to be whether or not to tell your employer. There are some pros and cons to this particular issue – the pros being that if some time in the future you have to file a claim for disability, it is on your work record that you suffer from chronic pain. Also if there is harassment or discrimination in the workplace based on disability, the workplace has been informed of your disability prior to the complaint being made. The cons are a fear of lack of advancement opportunities if a disability is disclosed, and some co-workers are uncomfortable about how to work with or treat people with disabilities.

The workplace and its equipment should be appropriate for the job and matched to the worker's disabilities. Sitting in an office chair and working at a desk were discussed earlier in this chapter under Sitting (see pages 66–67). As with household tasks, when muscles are used repeatedly or when they are required to hold a position for any length of time, they will fatigue, and so it is important to get up and move frequently (every 20–30 minutes), if your primary position is to sit at a desk all day. Intersperse your desk duties with tasks that involve standing, such as photocopying or filing. See your workplace Health and Safety Officer who can arrange for an occupational therapist to assess your workstation to meet your needs. Take adequate breaks, get away from your desk at morning coffee, lunchtime and teatime, and go for a walk around the exterior of the office, or maybe there is a park nearby where you can eat your lunch and relax. If you are a manual worker involved in lifting heavy items, there is a belt that can be bought from pharmacies to give support to the back muscles. This may be of assistance when lifting. Consider sharing the lifting with someone else to assess whether this makes the task easier for you. If you risk aggravating your pain further, ask to be relieved of lifting duties and offer to do other duties that you can do comfortably. Follow your local At Work Health and Safety Regulations.

Strict government legislation and regulations exist that employers must comply with in order to prevent people being killed, injured or contracting an illness in the workplace during workplace activities or due to specified high plant risk. As a result, many businesses and organisations employ workplace Health and Safety Officers to provide advice about workplace health and safety issues. They carry out inspections, set up educational programmes about workplace ealth and safety, help to investigate work injuries, work-caused illnesses and dangerous events.

Being involved in workplace rush hours (i.e. getting to work and leaving work) can put extra stress on people trying to manage their chronic pain. Have you ever thought about flexible working hours that allow you to travel to work outside the peak hours? Easing the stress allows you to arrive at work calmer and ready to pace yourself through the day. Flexible working hours can also mean reducing the hours you are currently working. Is it possible you could job-share with another person wanting to work part-time?

Equal opportunity legislation allows people not to be discriminated against because of their disability, age, race or gender. Many companies now have Personnel Departments, Occupational Health Departments or Equal Opportunities Officers, to ensure that discrimination does not take place within the workplace, and that the disabled employee is properly supported.

Some people in the workplace, particularly in small businesses where the numbers employed are few, are not aware of the Acts designed to protect workers' rights within the workplace. If workers are aware of the legislation they may choose not to use it because they fear losing their job if they complain to their employer about any of these issues. However, workers should be empowered to exercise their rights in the issues of health, safety and discrimination in the workplace. Your local Citizens Advice Bureau should be able to to give you relevant advice.

If you are unable to do your current job because of pain, have you considered retraining for another position within the same company? Maybe this is something to discuss with the Personnel Officer before giving up your employment. If your employer is unable to offer you retraining, you may need to consider contacting the Citizens Advice Bureau to ascertain what they are able to advise.

Perhaps you are unable to attend work like you used to do, as your pain has made it impossible to continue. If this is the case and you still need to earn an income, consultancy or freelance work, where you work from home, may be another option. Undertaking the latter allows you to work at your own pace and set your own deadlines. You can also fit in your own exercise programme or relaxation between tasks. There are books available about setting up a consultancy and working from home that can be purchased at bookshops or borrowed from your local library.

It may be that because of your pain you have been out of the workforce for some time but now feel you are able to return but need help settling back in. Your local job centre may be able to help you in this regard.

Many of the gadgets referred to in this chapter may be accessed through your occupational therapist or purchased at your local chemist or independent living centre. The latter and other similar retail outlets may be found in the Yellow Pages under "Disability – Information" or "Mobility – Access and Equipment".

CHAPTER SEVEN

EMOTIONAL SELF-HELP

When you are in pain, how well do you adapt to the situation? Do you mentally give in to the pain? Do you start feeling sorry for yourself and go to bed for the day, or do you fight the pain, getting frustrated and angry that the pain has disrupted your plans? No doubt, we have all given in to a headache at some time in our lives, taken a couple of paracetamol and gone for a lie down hoping the headache will have gone when we get up. Sometimes rest will remove pain, but it is usually acute pain, rather than chronic pain. For those who experience pain daily in their lives, lying down and feeling sorry for yourself is not going to fix the problem. Learning how to handle the emotions is a major factor in assisting in the management of chronic pain.

Anyone who has experienced chronic pain will have been through a rollercoaster ride of emotions (anger, guilt, sadness, depression) as they battle through the grief processes of a changed lifestyle, while trying to accept and come to terms with the changes. Frustration, as you try to find your physical and mental boundaries, is a feeling experienced by many when initially diagnosed with chronic pain. Prior to the pain, you might have been able to clean the house in a day, plus do the shopping and pay the bills. Now, however, it seems physically taxing to make the bed and just as mentally demanding to get the ingredients out of the cupboard to cook the evening meal. Frustration tends to lead to anger and all too often this anger is directed at family and friends because you think they are unable to understand what you are going through. This often results in loss of friendships, as friends no longer know how to relate to you and your moods. Talking through the issues and feelings involved can clear up a lot of misunderstandings that happen when people get frustrated or angry.

Family emotions are very much the same as yours (i.e. frustration, anger, guilt). Initially the family was increasingly attentive; they gave you a good deal of support and did more tasks around the home to help you get better. However, when the pain does not improve, the family's patience may begin to wear thin as they begin to resent the extra burden they have been handed. They withdraw from the immediate situation and get on with their own lives, which means you do not receive as much attention or assistance.

Expectations – yours and theirs – really help the process of managing pain if you are aware of your own personal limits. When you know this information, you can meet your own expectations of self and also address the expectations of others. People in chronic pain from time to time give excuses in answer to another's requests or expectations. As a person with chronic pain, you often need to check, when giving an excuse, to see if it is legitimate and not because you wish to avoid answering the request or expectation due to laziness, guilt, fear or being defiant to the request.

Guilt associated with the inability to do things for the family is often felt by the person experiencing chronic pain, whether it be due to no longer earning the family's income, or being unable to play sport with the teenagers in the family. Guilt often leads the person with chronic pain to do things that he or she knows will exacerbate the pain, because he or she has not dealt with the issue of guilt. This issue needs honest, straightforward communication between family and friends. For example, it is okay to let the younger children know you are no longer able to give them piggyback rides. Offer them an alternative such as building models with their Lego blocks or reading a story. By offering an alternative, you are keeping the channels of communication open for the children to request things of you in the future.

While others may know of your chronic pain, they may sometimes forget and make requests of you that push you further into the pain cycle. Being assertive allows you to not feel guilty because you have to refuse a request, although being assertive does not always mean saying no. Assertiveness is being able to say what you think and allowing others to do the same. Being assertive is almost impossible when your self-esteem and confidence are low. Ask someone to help you talk with your family (e.g. clergy, friend, relative, professional counsellor), but don't leave it too late to address the problem. To improve your assertive skills, you could attend a course in assertiveness training offered at many evening classes. If you feel some one-to-one counselling is needed in preference to the group situation of joining a course, seek out a professional counsellor, such as a psychologist or social worker. Your family doctor may also be able to recommend an independent counsellor.

Achieving is a self-help way of improving self-esteem. Start out by setting yourself a small and realistic goal – something you want to do and will enjoy. Keep telling yourself that you are a competent and capable person and that you are going to succeed. This positive self-talk will motivate you and rebuild your confidence. The goal need not be a financial one. A great deal of self-satisfaction can be gained by helping others. Many voluntary organisations could use one or two hours of your time. Remember that kindness costs nothing but you reap huge rewards when you think of others, and have less inclination to worry about yourself.

There is a tendency to socially withdraw from others when self-esteem is low and confidence is lacking. However, this issue needs to be dealt with quickly because if it is not addressed, it can lead to social isolation. This may lead you into a downward spiral until there are feelings of sadness and depression that things aren't the same as they used to be. It is not unusual at this stage, that some may even consider suicide as a way out of their predicament. Depression is a grief reaction to changed circumstances, which usually involves loss (e.g. loss of a limb, loss of a previous lifestyle etc.). There are degrees of depression. There is usually enough support in the family to deal with mild episodes of depression, but severe depression, where you consider life no longer worth living, calls for the need to see your family doctor for professional intervention and treatment, or referral to a specialist.

Acceptance of chronic pain is probably the most difficult step of all but the most important, because it allows you to get on with your life. Acceptance is not only acknowledging that you are in pain, but that while you are experiencing pain, high physical and mental demands on yourself are quite unrealistic. Acceptance enables you to adapt your lifestyle to make the necessary changes for you to be as comfortable as you can. You learn to adapt through time. Adaptation is about pacing yourself to what you reasonably can do when in pain. For example, it is no good planning to weed the garden or vacuum the house when it is a day your pain is bad. Pacing yourself is not just giving in to pain; it is finding a comfortable alternative. Instead of weeding the garden or vacuuming, you catch up on bill paying by telephone, or letter writing to friends or some mending from the workbasket. Set yourself realistic goals that can be achieved.

Modern day approaches in assisting people with chronic pain tend to assess the person's attitude towards having pain (i.e. what are their thoughts and feelings about their pain?). Pain can result in having a negative mindset and make a person cranky and irritable with others. This negative mindset gives a 'victim mentality' which leads to a 'poor me' attitude being exhibited. This is a road to nowhere with very little respect for yourself or from others. The idea is to understand attitude as a state of mind that can be controlled. By changing your mindset to having a positive attitude, you can change so many aspects of your life. Having a positive attitude shows:

- You respect yourself, which flows on to others to show you respect
- You are accepting of change
- You have good self-esteem and confidence
- You are able to be assertive
- You are in control of your emotions

A positive attitude not only involves positive thoughts but also positive behaviours. Behaviours that make you feel good about yourself include pleasurable activities (e.g. visiting a neighbour and taking morning tea or having a neighbour visit you for morning tea). Positive attitude just doesn't happen overnight; it is a challenge for you to work on every day, so that you adapt to your changed lifestyle much more quickly.

Affirmations are techniques by which you can change negative thoughts to positive ones. They are used in autogenic training. Using these techniques allows you to overcome thoughts and feelings of negativity that accompany chronic pain. For example, a negative thought might be, 'Pain makes me anxious.' An affirmation to counteract the negative thought might be, 'I will relax and trust others.' Repetition of an affirmation has a self-hypnotic effect, so by often repeating the positive statement to yourself, you can combat the negative thought or feeling. Put your affirmations where you can see them (e.g. on the fridge door or bathroom mirror.) Your affirmations can be unique to you, although a lot of people use the 'Serenity' prayer, which in simple translation means, 'Learn to accept the things you cannot change and stop wasting valuable energy worrying about things and wishing things were different.'

Some people experiencing pain, particularly if they are not coping well with their pain, have found it helpful to keep a journal that they fill with daily thoughts and feelings on how their day has gone. The journal is usually filled in each evening reflecting the day's events. Self-analysis takes place to ascertain whether you could do something better should similar events or feelings happen in the future.

Anxiety is usually concerned with worries about the future or fears of the unknown. People with chronic pain are susceptible to anxiety – for example, fear of the unknown where a doctor prescribes a certain medical procedure without providing the full details about it. To resolve your anxiety, gather enough information on which to make an informed decision to dispense some of the anxiety before submitting to any procedure. Fear of the future can make today miserable, particularly when we do not know what is around the corner. Live for today. Tomorrow will take care of itself. Use affirmations when you first get up in the morning to tell yourself you are going to have a good day and mean it.

Worrying constantly causes you to be tense and tension inevitably leads to fatigue. Unfortunately, fatigue exacerbates pain levels, not to mention making you cranky and irritable. If you are a constant worrier, set aside 10 minutes each day to address your worries, but not before bedtime when you want to be relaxed to go to sleep. During this time write down one or two concerns and brainstorm one or two solutions for each of them, then choose a solution to solve the worry. Remember that you can only make decisions for what you will do for yourself. Leave others to make their own decisions.

CHAPTER EIGHT

PRACTICAL SELF-HELP

Throughout this book, much emphasis has beeplaced on the importance of calming the body and mind as a method of alleviating or reducing pain levels. This chapter concentrates on the different types of relaxation you can adopt to help you manage your pain. It is important to note, however, that some methods are more physically active than others, so only practise a method that is suitable to your own needs.

Once again the topic has been addressed alphabetically, not because one method is better than another, but because it is often easier to find when listed alphabetically. Let's start off with the most important aspect of calming the mind and body – breathing.

BREATHING

Breathing is taught to pregnant women to help them breathe their way through the pain of labour. Paramedics and ambulance personnel on arriving at the scene of an accident will often instruct the patient to take deep breaths as a method of calming the patient down, if the patient is distressed and/or experiencing pain.

Most people are shallow breathers in that they breathe in only as far as their chest and breathe out through their mouth. Deep breathing is where you slowly breathe in to fill the lungs, breathing deeper and slower to fill the abdomen also. Just as slowly, you breathe out to expel the air. When done properly this has a calming, relaxing effect on the body and mind. Deep breathing takes practice, as anyone who has engaged in Tai Chi or yoga will tell you. The best time to practise is first thing in the morning and in bed before you go to sleep.

To practise deep breathing, first lie comfortably on your back, putting the palms of your hands, with fingertips touching, across your abdomen. You will notice when breathing out that your fingertips will touch and when breathing in that your fingertips will part. It is important to breathe out as slowly as you breathe in. As you become more accomplished at deep breathing, you will find you are able to breathe more deeply and while you have learned the method lying down, you will be able to put the deep breathing technique into practice when sitting or standing. The response to this calmly relaxed feeling may eliminate pain or reduce its intensity.

As an adjunct to breathing, the technique of centring eliminates the occupied mind, and allows it to relax. Close your eyes, either sitting or lying down, and bring awareness to your breathing. Inhale slowly and deeply, preferably with your mouth closed, so that you can feel the air passing through your nostrils. Close your mind to now, think only of the creation of a third eye in the middle of your forehead – concentrating on the third eye position in the middle of your forehead allows you to be centred and for the mind to eliminate other thoughts. Some people find it useful to say a single word or mantra to stop their mind from wandering. If thoughts come into your head, do not judge them but let them pass, always bringing your awareness back to the third eye. Centring can take anything around 5–20 minutes. The more practice you give to this method, the quicker your mind will empty.

The body also needs to relax, so try to combine deep muscle relaxation with breathing. You should allow 20–30 minutes for this type of relaxation. Firstly find a comfortable location where you are unlikely to be disturbed. Take the telephone off the hook, use a fan or music to blot out any background noise. Practise deep muscle relaxation before you eat, rather than after. Loosen any tight clothing and take off your shoes, glasses, watch or jewellery. Make a decision not to worry about anything. Give your mind and body this time to heal. This is your time.

Commence by lying down on a bed, a carpet or sitting in a chair. Start your slow deep breathing and on the out breath, imagine any tension in your body flowing away. Start this exercise at the feet. Tense your feet, point them downwards, and stretch them as far as you can. Hold the stretch for seven to ten seconds then release, letting your feet flop to the sides. Continue breathing slowly. Next go to your calf muscles and tense them by stretching for seven to ten seconds (take care not to overstretch if you are susceptible to cramps in this region, although the slow deep breathing will help to protect against cramps). Then let go, relaxing the muscles for 10–15 seconds. Next tense your hips and thighs for seven to ten seconds. Feel the stretch then relax, feeling these body parts go heavy as the muscles relax. Next squeeze the buttocks together. Hold the squeeze for seven to ten seconds then let go. Next tighten the stomach muscles and arch your back if you do not suffer lower back pain. Hold the pose for seven to ten seconds and then relax. Next tighten your chest wall for seven to ten seconds. Slowly breathe out and relax. Next, squeeze your hands shut into fists and imagine you are squeezing the juice from a lemon. When you have squeezed your hardest imagine dropping the lemon by opening your hands and letting go. Next tense the arms by stretching downwards, trying to reach your toes. Then let go. Next tense your shoulders by pushing them upwards towards your ears. How far will your chin come down to meet your shoulders? Hold the pose for seven to ten seconds then relax and let go. Finally, screw up your face by clenching your eyelids shut and opening your mouth as far as you can. Relax. Keep your eyes closed and allow your jaw to go limp. Let your head settle itself where it will, then feel the peace. Enjoy the calm atmosphere that is invading your body for the next 10–15 minutes.

As you come out of deep relaxation, blink your eyes a few times and then lift your body slowly into the sitting position, if you have been lying down, to relax. If you experience pain that is below the waist you may wish to do the relaxation exercise in reverse, starting at the head and going down to your feet.

GUIDED IMAGERY OR VISUALISATION

Guided imagery or visualisation can be a powerful tool to reduce or eliminate pain. It is another form of relaxation for the body and mind. Guided imagery or visualisation involves using the mind to calm the tension pain is causing in your body. Possibly the easiest type of imagery or visualisation to start with is that of associating shapes and colours to your pain. Let's say you are having a bad day with pain. Concentrate on the area your pain is in and think of a colour that describes your current level of pain. If your pain is tingling or has a burning sensation, you may put the colours of red or orange to your pain. Or if your pain is dull and aching, you may imagine the colour to be black or grey. How can you change the intensity of your pain through colour? Think of a colour that you find calming and cool to counteract the burning sensation or throbbing that you feel. Perhaps visualise a blue or green, then in your mind transfer this colour to the area of your pain. Concentrate on the coolness and calmness of the colour to the area as you breathe to relax the mind and body. Think of things in calming colours – for example, the soft blue calm of the ocean, the clear blue of the sky on a sunny day and the green of the countryside after fresh rain.

The same imagery can be done with shapes. For example, the shape of your pain on a bad day may be like jagged broken glass or pointed like the blade of a knife. Think of an alternative shape that can be relaxing. Some people consider the waves of the ocean relaxing. Concentrate on the wavy lines and guide the image to the area of pain. After 5–10 minutes you should feel the pain reducing. Others think of weight on a bad day when the pain is heavy and feel they are dragging themselves around. Change this thought to something light, such as fluffy white clouds floating across the sky.

O. Carl Simonton (detailed in his book, *Getting Well Again: A step-by-step, self-help guide to overcoming cancer for patients and their families*) used visual imagery with cancer patients. He had the patients visualise their bodies as a computer game, similar to Pac-Man. They had to visualise the little 'Pac-Men' eating up the cancer cells in their bodies and leaving only the healthy cells so that they would get well again. It was found that, on average, cancer patients that had used visualisation techniques lived twice as long as other cancer patients.

Visualisation also extends to visualising places that you find relaxing. For some people it may be the beach with the sound of waves gently lapping the shore and the pleasant heat of the sun on your body. For others it may be the coolness and quiet of the rainforest with a trickling stream splashing water over small rocks. This visualising of place can be as short or as long a relaxation session as you wish it to be. Preparing for the time to relax is the same as centring and deep muscle relaxation, although the script is different. To carry out guided imagery or visualisation, first become comfortable with your eyes closed. If not, place yourself in a comfortable position.

To begin, commence deep breathing. Visualise that you are walking along a country road, the sun is shining and you feel warm and relaxed. You hear the crunch of gravel under your feet. You see a path taking you off the road into a green meadow. Take the path to the bottom of the meadow. Climb over the small wall at the bottom of the meadow – this leads you into a copse of trees. Follow the pathway into a small wood of trees. Visualise the changes from the meadow. Notice the sun is not as strong and is dappled on the pathway as it shines through the trees. The temperature has changed. It is cooler than the meadow. There is a damp smell of wet leaves on the floor of the copse and you can hear the sound of a bird as it calls out to its mate amongst the trees. Continue walking, enjoying the feelings of solitude and peace. The trees are getting thicker and you can hear the sound of running water. You continue walking, noticing that every so often the scene is changing – there are now small rocks between the trees and on the sides of the pathway. The sound of water is coming closer. It is a splashing sound. The trees are opening out a little at a time and you come to a pool. Looking across the pool of water you see bigger rocks and hear the sound of water as it splashes over the rocks into the pool. There is a tree stump that looks worn at the side of the pool on which you sit down. You pick up a tiny stone to toss into the pool. Imagine the tiny stone is your pain. As you watch the ripple get bigger, follow the circles in your mind's eye. The circles are taking your pain away. Enjoy the peace and pleasantness of the scene. Rest and relax and stay in this visualisation for as long as you can. Now come out of the relaxation slowly so as not to disturb the inner peace you are feeling.

There are many different scripts for many different places, from the beach to the rainforest. Initially when you begin guided imagery or visualisation as a relaxation method, you may need someone to talk you through a scene. A psychologist or nurse could probably do this for you and provide you with a tape recording of their voice that you can use in your home as you practise this method of relaxation. Alternatively you could put your own visualisations onto a tape and play it as you relax. As you become adept at using this method, you will find you don't need verbal prompts, and you can visualise in silence or listening to soft music.

LEISURE

The Oxford Dictionary defines leisure as having free time at one's own disposal, which suggests this is a time for doing something that is enjoyable. There are many benefits to be gained by having an interest and taking time out for leisure activities. These activities provide a form of relaxation, a way of socialising, a way to override pain where new skills are learnt and confidence is gained. Pleasurable pastimes can distract us from pain because concentration is placed on the activity, leaving no time to think about pain. By retaining or developing an interest or carrying out leisure activities you have something to talk about to others as well as having a focus for your life other than pain.

Local communities offer a great range of activities; whether it be volunteering in something you enjoy (e.g. drama class, choral group, charity work), learning a new skill, taking time to read a book and improve your knowledge and gain inspiration (e.g. local library), being creative and doing craft work (e.g. making the family's Christmas or birthday presents), or simply socialising in local pubs or community centres.

Others find that they prefer to do their leisure activities at home, particularly if they are experiencing feelings of anger about their pain. I know of one young person who finds relief in doing mosaics. She obtains relief from anger by productively smashing ceramic tiles for her mosaics, and finds it soothing artistically to place the broken ceramic tiles into a mosaic pattern. Another person visually relaxes when she is at her pottery wheel shaping clay.

Initially, try to choose a couple of pleasurable activities that you can do over the week. Choose one active and one passive activity, as this will allow you flexibility on days when your pain is bothering you. Make time in your weekly schedule to pursue your leisure activities and remember to pace yourself.

MASSAGE

You can get pain relief from massage and while some people like to use a masseuse or a physiotherapist for massage, it is also something you can do for yourself. I learnt a wonderful self-massage technique for my back pain at a yoga class. It involves lying on the carpet and bringing your knees up to your chest. Hug your knees with your hands and arms. Gently start to rotate the bottom of your back in a small circular motion. As you progress make the circles bigger, covering a larger area of your back. Then, as you finish your self-massage, make the circles smaller again. 5–10 minutes of this massage can help relieve aches and pains for some people.

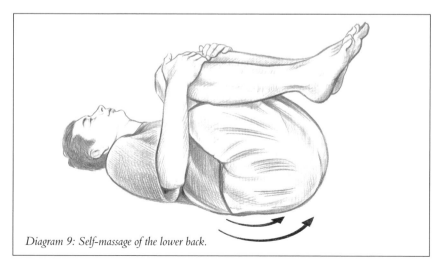

Diagram 9: Self-massage of the lower back.

MEDITATION

What are the benefits of meditation? There is a decrease in stress-related physical problems such as high blood pressure, palpitations, insomnia, stuttering and tension headaches. Meditation eases tension and anxiety. Meditation increases the feelings of peace and self-worth and it allows for the emotional release of negative feelings. Sitting in meditation, silent and still, watching thoughts come and go, can bring peace of mind. Meditation allows us to switch off the pressure of the busy lives we lead.

When practising meditation, try to find a peaceful location in the home where there are no distractions or disturbances. Many people who meditate do so early in the morning before the other occupant(s) of the house are awake. They find that this prepares them for their day ahead. Others like to meditate when they arrive home from work, thereby taking time for themselves before they change their role of breadwinner to family member. Others may meditate last thing at night to create a peaceful mind on which to sleep. If you wish, an aromatic candle or an incense stick can be lit to sweeten the vibrations. The light of the candle can also give you something to focus on as you meditate. Once you have found your ideal location and the time of day when meditation is most agreeable with you, keep them regular as familiarity will make it easier to slip into your calming routine.

The traditional posture for meditation is sitting on a cushion with your legs crossed. If your legs are flexible, you can try tucking one of your crossed legs under the other and having the leg that is crossed on top turned, so that the sole of the foot is in an upward position. In yoga, this position is known as the half lotus.

Some people find it useful to have a mantra to meditate on. They choose a word such as 'relax' or 'peace' to create a relaxation response. Others prefer a spiritual word such as 'shalom' or 'Hail Mary', as part of their meditation ritual.

If you are not able to sit on the floor, then use a comfortable chair with your back relaxed against the back of it and your feet touching the floor. Do not get so comfortable that you may fall asleep, as it is essential to remain aware while the body rests. Rest your hands in your lap.

While sitting quietly doing nothing, the unwinding process will start to happen if you let it. Breathe normally and after each exhalation count to three and start breathing again. Let your thoughts come and go – this is not easy initially when the mind is hyperactive. A mantra can sometimes help the hyperactive mind. Choose a word such as 'relax' or 'peace' to get you back on track.

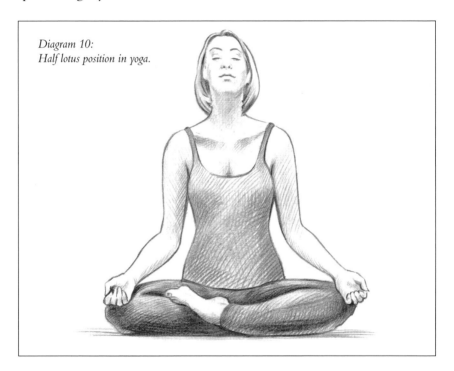

Diagram 10:
Half lotus position in yoga.

People ask how long they should do their meditation for. There is no need to watch the clock, as your body will let you know when you are ready to end the meditation. However, initially, aim for 15–20 minutes as you practise the technique. You will find your time extending as you become more comfortable with the physical posture and the quietening of the mind. Meditation provides us with a psychological breathing space; it centres us when we are stressed and creates a heightened awareness of our priorities in life. Learn to enjoy this time of solitude.

In coming out of meditation, try to keep the feelings of calm for as long as you can. Don't rush around trying to catch up feeling guilty for the time you have had to yourself. Get into the habit of slowing your life down.

PRAYER

In times of great stress many people, who would not normally consider themselves religious, turn to prayer as a means of addressing the unbearable tension they are going through. There are also the people who pray regularly and believe in the power of prayer. It makes no difference what faith you believe in – prayer encompasses all faiths. For some the 'Serenity' prayer is enough to ease their burdens, without the ritual of attending a church or mosque:

> *God give us the grace to accept with serenity the things that cannot be changed;*
> *Courage to change the things that should be changed;*
> *And the wisdom to distinguish one from the other.*
> Reinhold Niebuhr, 1932

Prayer can be a way of sharing one's pain, whether it is physical pain or the emotional aspects of pain such as grief and anxiety. What we pray for is unique to each of us, but it is a way of clarifying our thoughts and focussing on what is real to us. The physical structure of prayer is similar to that of relaxation. The quiet surroundings of a church or chapel, the soft organ music filling our senses, our closed eyes allowing us to withdraw from distractions around us. All of these things are similar to some of the relaxation methods discussed elsewhere in this chapter.

Many people find that prayer brings them inner peace, providing them with added strength to deal with their pain and stress. No one knows how spirituality affects health, although some experts attribute the healing effect to hope, which is known to benefit the immune system. Others liken spiritual acts and beliefs to meditation, which decreases muscle tension and can lower heart rates.

SELF-NURTURING

Self-nurturing means treating yourself with unconditional love or looking after yourself in the best way possible. Try to think back to when you last took part in any of the following relaxing activities:

- Drank a bottle of wine with dinner served in your nicest glass-ware (you can purchase non-alcoholic wine if alcohol cannot be used with your medication).
- Read a book or saw a movie that you would like to read or see (this pure escapism from everyday tasks can be enjoyable and fun).
- Soaked in a long luxurious bath with fragrant bath oils and bubbles (not only good for aches and pains but the aromas give you a feeling of peace and contentment).
- Walked on a beach as the sun was coming up or going down (apart from the exercise of walking, the scene is sure to provide you with a relaxed feeling).

Such small luxuries can bring about positive moods and feelings, which can enhance your immune system. The pleasure one feels when indulging in one or two of these little luxuries can distract your mind from pain. Treat yourself to a little luxury – do something for yourself today.

CONCLUSION

Chronic pain will not alter unless you are prepared to make changes to get the best quality out of life that you can. Throughout the book we have discussed the ingredients for change for those who experience chronic pain. Along with these ingredients, the following factors are also needed for change:

- Acceptance of what is passed. Once reached, acceptance puts a spring in your step and a sparkle in your eye. It's a chance to start afresh and make each day the best you can.
- An attitude of willingness to make changes to your lifestyle that give you comfort and pleasure.
- An open mind to new ideas and a plan of action starting now to encompass the ideas that appeal to you. Remember – small achievements lead to larger gains.

There is no such word as failure to the optimist. All that is needed is perseverance to try again. With these factors and patience on your side, you can live a better life.

ADDRESSES

British Chiropractic Association
Blagrave House
17 Blagrave Street
Reading
Berkshire
RG1 1QB
Tel: 0118 950 5950
Fax: 0118 958 8946
www.chiropractic-uk.co.uk

British Dietetic Association
5th Floor, Charles House
148/9 Great Charles Street
Queensway
Birmingham
B3 3HT
Tel: 0121 200 8080
Fax: 0121 200 8081
www.BDA.uk.com
Email: info@bda.uk.com

British Psychological Society
St Andrews House
48 Princess Road East
Leicester
LE1 7DR
Tel: 0116 254 9568
Fax: 0116 247 0787
www.bps.org.uk
Email: enquiry@bps.org.uk

Chartered Society of Physiotherapists (CSP)
(for list of physios)
      www.csp.org.uk/physio2u.cfm
      Email: physio2u.csp.org.uk

Citizens Advice Bureau
      www.citizensadvice.org.uk

College of Occupational Therapy
      Enquiry line: 0800 389 4873
      www.otipp.co.uk

NHS Self-Management Programme
(for further information)
      Tel: 01245 295 043
      Email:pete.moore@chelmsford-pcg.nhs.uk

Pain Society
      The Secretariat, The Pain Society
      21 Portland Place
      London W1B 1PY
      Tel: 020 7631 8870
      www.painsociety.org

Royal London Homeopathic Hospital
      60 Great Ormond Street
      London WC1N 3HR
      Tel: 020 7837 2880

Royal Pharmaceutical Society of Great Britain
      1 Lambeth High Street
      London SE1 7JN
      Tel: 020 7735 9141
      www.rpsgb.org.uk
      Email: enquiries@rpsgb.org.uk

REFERENCES

Barnard N., 1998, *Foods that Fight Pain*, Harmony Books, New York

Benjamin B.E. Borden G., 1984, *Listen to your Pain*, Viking Press, New York

Bogin M., 1982, *The Path to Pain Control*, Houghton Miffin & Co., Boston

Chaiatow L., 1995, *Fibromyalgia and Muscle Pain*, Thorsons, London

Devi N.J., 2000, *The Healing Path of Yoga*, Three Rivers Press, New York

Erlich Williamson M., 1996, *Fibromyalgia*, Allen & Unwin, Sydney

Erlich Williamson M., 1998, *The Fibromyalgia Relief Book*, Walker & Co., New York

Fontana D., 1991, *The Elements of Meditation*, Element, Shaftesbury

Gawler, I., 1996, *Meditation Pure and Simple*, Hill of Content, Melbourne

Goldberg P. (Ed.), 1997, *Pain Remedies: From Little Ouches to Big Aches*, Rodale Press Inc., Emmaus, Pennsylvania

Harte D.A., 1992, *Tai Chi Handbook* (2nd Edition), Trunkline Productions, Auckland

Hendler N., Fenton J., 1979, *Coping with Chronic Pain*, Clarkson N. Potter Inc, New York

Jayson M.I. & I.V., 1987, *Back Pain: The Facts*, Oxford University Press, Oxford

Kittredge M., 1992, 'Pain', *Encyclopaedia of Health*, Chelsea House, New York

Linchitz R.M., *Life without Pain*, Addison Wesley Publishing Co. Inc., Reading, Massachusetts

Masters, P., 1988, *Osteopathy for Everyone*, Penguin, London

McIlwain H.H., Fulghum Bruce D., 1996, *The Fibromyalgia Handbook*, Henry Holt, New York

McGill I., 1997, *The Chiropractors Health Book*, Crown Trade Paperbacks, New York

Melzack R., Wall P., 1983, *The Challenge of Pain*, Basic Book Inc., New York

Li, Ding, 1988, *Transmitting Qi along the Meridian: Meridian Qigong*, Foreign Language Press, Beijing

Nardo D. (Garrell D. Ed.), 1992, *Medical Diagnosis*, Chelsea House, New York

Nicholas M., Molloy A., Tonkin L., Beeston L., 2000, *Manage Your Pain*, ABC Books, Sydney

Norfolk D., 1986, *Conquering Back Pain*, Blandford Press, Dorset

Nottidge P., Lamphugh D., 1974, *Stress and Overstress*, Angus & Robertson, London

Occupational Therapy Department, 1998, *Back Care in Daily Living Tasks*, District Health Service Bundaberg

Pawlett R., 2001, *A Beginner's Guide to Shiatsu*, D&S Books, Bideford

Pelleteir, K., 2000, *The Best Alternative Medicine*, Simon & Schuster, New York

Proto L., 1986, *How to Beat Fatigue*, Century Arrow, London

Readers Digest, 1992, *Guide to Alternative Medicine*, Readers Digest, Sydney

Reicheimer S., 2000, *New Technologies for Treating Back Pain and Sciatica*, Reicheimer Pain Institute, Los Angeles

Shaw J Ed., 1990, *The Australian Medical Association Guide to Medicine and Drugs*, Readers Digest, Sydney

Simonton, O. Carl, Matthews-Simonton, S, & Greighton, James, L., 1980, *Getting Well Again: A Step-by-Step, Self-help Guide to overcoming cancer for patients and their families.* Bantam Books, Toronto.

Stewart A., 1993, *Tired all the Time*, Vermillion, London

Sternbach R., 1987, *Mastering Pain: A Twelve Step Regimen for Coping with Chronic Pain*, Arlington Books, London

Swanson D. W. (Ed), 1999, *Mayo Clinic on Chronic Pain*, Kensington Publishing, New York

Wallace L. M., 1990, *Coping with Angina*, Thorsons, Wellingborough

Young, J., 1994, *Acupressure for Health*, Thorsons, London

INDEX